THE ULTIMATE
GIRLS' BODY BOOK

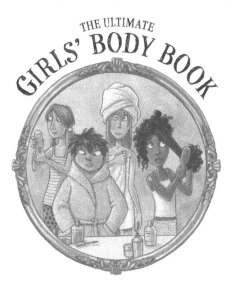

Praise for The Ultimate Girls' Body Book

In my personal research, I have not found a more comprehensive and useful resource for young women looking to understand their bodies. *The Ultimate Girls' Body Book* removes the opportunity for misunderstandings or lack of information that could handicap a girl for life. I'm eager and delighted for both my daughters to have a copy to study with me.

> —*Jennie Bishop, author of* The Princess and the Kiss *and* Planned Purity
> for Parents, *founder of PurityWorks, Daytona Beach, Florida*

Dr. Walt and Dr. Wohlever have written a thoughtful guide for tween girls and their parents that is scientifically sound, biblically grounded, and entirely practical. They answer the questions that everyone is too embarrassed to talk about.

> —*Julian T. Hsu, MD, family physician, assistant clinical professor,*
> *University of Colorado Health Sciences Center, Denver, Colorado*

The Ultimate Girls' Body Book is an amazing resource for parents. We are grateful that a trusted medical professional has taken the time to write this much-needed guide for girls. Dr. Walt Larimore is a unique combination of medical expert, outstanding communicator, and compassionate advisor. He uses those gifts to lead young readers through the often-puzzling journey of adolescence by answering the questions they are often afraid to voice.

> —*Mark Merrill, president of Family First and author of* All Pro Dad
> —*Susan Merrill, founder and director of iMOM.com and author of*
> The Passionate Mom

This book is fun and approachable. It is written with sensitivity, yet it is also realistic and direct. This is something a tween can relate to. I am picky about books, but this is a wonderful resource that can serve as a valuable guidepost for families with tween girls. I plan to recommend it to family and friends.

> —*Ann Park, MD, women's development coach and founder of*
> *CoachingwithDrAnn.com, Tampa, Florida*

Other Writings by the Authors

By Walt Larimore, MD

Nonfiction Books

The Ultimate Guys' Body Book:
Not-So-Stupid Questions About Your Body

Lintball Leo's Not-So-Stupid Questions About Your Body

10 Essentials of Happy, Healthy People:
Becoming and Staying Highly Healthy

Alternative Medicine: The Christian Handbook

SuperSized Kids: How to Rescue Your Child
from the Obesity Threat

Why A.D.H.D. Doesn't Mean Disaster

His Brain, Her Brain: How Divinely Designed
Differences Can Strengthen Your Marriage

The Honeymoon of Your Dreams:
A Practical Guide to Planning a Romantic Honeymoon

Workplace Grace: Becoming a Spiritual Influence at Work

Workplace Grace: Becoming a Spiritual Influence at Work —
Groupware™ Curriculum
(Includes video, DVD, leader's guide, and participant's workbook)

Grace Prescriptions: Becoming a Spiritual Influence
in Healthcare
(Small-group curriculum with leader's guide and participant's workbook;
coauthored with William Carr Peel)

*The Saline Solution: Becoming a Spiritual Influence
in Your Medical Practice*
(Small-group curriculum with DVD, leader's guide, and participant's
workbook; coauthored with William Carr Peel)

Autobiographical Books

*Bryson City Tales: Stories of a Doctor's First Year of Practice
in the Smoky Mountains*

*Bryson City Seasons: More Tales of a Doctor's Practice in
the Smoky Mountains*

*Bryson City Secrets: Even More Tales of a Small-Town
Doctor in the Smoky Mountains*

Novels

Time Series Investigators: The Gabon Virus

Time Series Investigators: The Influenza Bomb
(coauthored with Paul McCusker)

Hazel Creek: A Novel

Sugar Fork: A Novel

Websites

Dr. Walt's website is www.DrWalt.com.

Dr. Walt's health blog is www.DrWalt.com/blog.

*Purchase autographed books at
www.Dr-Walts-store.hostedbyamazon.com.*

*Morning Glory, Evening Grace Daily Devotional,
available at www.Devotional.DrWalt.com*

By Amaryllis Sánchez Wohlever, MD

Nonfiction Books

Walking with Jesus in Healthcare: A 120-day devotional to refresh your soul as you care for others

Bible commentary published in The Journey

Faith in Action: Living a Life of Blessing
(a study of James and the Beatitudes)

Marks of the Kingdom (based on the Gospel According to Matthew)

Prayer in the Early Church (based on Acts of the Apostles)

The Radiance of God's Glory (a study of the book of Hebrews)

Turning Points of the Faith

Study of the Gospel According to Mark

Studies of Paul's Letters (Philippians, 1 Corinthians,
1 and 2 Thessalonians)

Study of Letters of Peter, John, and Jude

Websites

Dr. Mari's blog is www.DrMarisFaithStop.com.

Dr. Mari's author website is www.faithfulmd.wordpress.com.

Dr. Mari writes devotions for Good News Daily *and* Bible commentary *for* The Journey
(published by Bible Reading Fellowship — www.biblereading.org)

Learn about Dr. Mari's writing, editing, and Spanish translations at www.DrMarisFaithStop.com.

Not-So-Silly Questions
About Your Body

THE ULTIMATE GIRLS' BODY BOOK

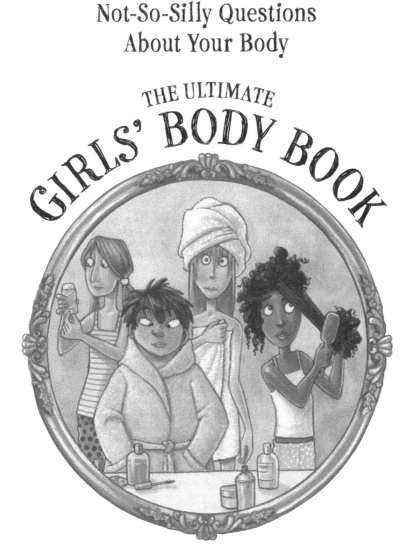

Walt Larimore, MD
Amaryllis Sánchez Wohlever, MD

ZONDERkidz

ZONDERKIDZ

The Ultimate Girls' Body Book
Copyright © 2013 by Dr. Walt Larimore and Dr. Amaryllis Sánchez Wohlever

This title is also available as a Zondervan ebook.
Visit www.zondervan.com/ebooks

Requests for information should be addressed to:
Zonderkidz, 5300 Patterson Ave SE, Grand Rapids, Michigan 49530

Library of Congress Cataloging-in-Publication Data

Larimore, Walter L.
    Not-so-silly questions about your body : the ultimate girls' body book /
Walt Larimore, MD, and Amaryllis Sánchez Wohlever, MD.
        pages cm.
    Audience: 9–12.
    ISBN 978-0-310-73981-4 (softcover)
    1. Teenage girls—Health and hygiene—Juvenile literature. 2. Beauty,
Personal—Religious aspects—Christianity—Juvenile literature. 3. Human
body—Religious aspects—Christianity—Juvenile literature. I. Wohlever,
Amaryllis Sanchez. II. Title. III. Title: Ultimate girls' body book.
RA777.25.L37 2013
    613'.0433—dc23   2013027953

The content in a number of the chapters in this book (2, 3, 5, 6, 11, 19, 20, 24, 25, 26,
29, 31, 32, 33, 34) has been heavily adapted, with permission from ZonderKidz, from
The Ultimate Guys' Body Book: Not-So-Stupid Questions About Your Body, © 2012
by Dr. Walt Larimore. The poem quoted by the woman in Question 3 ("The Hidden
Masterpiece") is adapted from Grant Colfax Tullar's poem "The Weaver". The story
of the Lopez family in Question 11 is adapted from www.SuperSizedKids.com with
the permission of Florida Hospital Publishing in Orlando, FL.

Cover design: Cindy Davis
Interior illustration: Guy Francis
Editor: Kim Childress
Interior composition: Greg Johnson/Textbook Perfect

Printed in the United States of America

14 15 16 17 18 19 /QVS/ 18 17 16 15 14 13 12 11 10 9 8 7 6 5 4 3 2 1

For Anna Katherine and Sarah Elisabeth
May you always be as beautiful on the inside as you are
on the outside.

Pop

For Hannah, whose pure heart and love of God will
forever make her beautiful.
And for Mami, whose legacy of love lives on.

A.S.W.

Disclaimer

This book contains advice and information relating to health and medicine. It is designed for your personal knowledge and to help you be a more informed consumer of medical and health services. It is not intended to be exhaustive or to replace medical advice from your physician and should be used to supplement rather than replace regular care by your physician. Readers should consult their physicians with specific questions and concerns. All efforts have been made to ensure the accuracy of the information contained within this book.

CONTENTS

This book is enhanced with QR codes that link to valuable articles and websites. Look for these codes throughout the book.

NOTE TO PARENTS

The Ultimate Girls' Body Book was written to help equip girls and the adults who love them during the change-packed years of puberty. We know it can be tough to approach subjects like their changing bodies, moods, and the world of boy-girl relationships. So we've provided conversation starters to help you embrace this time of change, learn together, and enjoy the journey.

Puberty means body changes, acne, and menstrual periods. It means talks about hormones, boys, and sex. It also means texts, phone calls, slumber parties and, yes, more texts. No worries. This book will help you talk about all this and raise a healthy daughter. You can reassure her that puberty is a normal, God-designed process that helps her transition from girl to woman. Your loving guidance will make all the difference.

As Christian family doctors, we want you to have accurate medical information that is biblically sound. So we reviewed the latest research and national guidelines through the lens of a biblical worldview. We also had every chapter reviewed by the Christian Medical Association and researchers, physicians, dietitians, psychologists, coaches, educators, and mom-daughter teams (they're listed under Acknowledgments).

Let us share a word of caution. We care deeply about preserving your daughter's innocence and know she may not be ready for certain topics. Yet, we can't ignore the dangers that lurk in a broken world. The latter part of the book contains more mature subjects. Help guide her reading and stay engaged. Decide which topics should wait. You know her best.

We recommend that you read the book together. Be available for discussions while cooking dinner or driving to school, at the mall or during nightly walks. A simple question like, *What did you think about the chapter on friendship?* may open a door to new ways of relating. Reading together will make it easier to establish healthy boundaries for your family.

Another option is to read the book on your own first. If it seems appropriate for her maturity level, let her read it. But be intentional. Keep track of her progress and give her opportunities to ask questions. You won't have all the answers, but you can show her you care by sharing the journey.

Consider journaling about your feelings and questions. Share your awkward puberty stories and laugh. Pray together and have fun. The seeds you plant now will bear fruit for a lifetime.

> Start children off on the way they should go, and even when they are old they will not turn from it.
>
> *Proverbs 22:6*

NOTE TO GIRLS

Welcome to puberty! *To what?* Yes! You're near or smack in the middle of the exciting (and puzzling!) time called *puberty*. Do you like roller coasters? Awesome! Buckle your seatbelt as you learn all about God's plan to grow you from girl to young woman.

You may wonder, *When will I start wearing a bra and shaving my legs? And what on earth are periods?* We'll answer your questions and make you laugh too. You'll learn about dealing with pimples and what true beauty is all about. We'll talk about your changing body, liking boys, texting, bullies, and more.

Read this book with your mom or another trusted woman. Choose fun spots to chat with her about all you're learning. Talk while painting your toenails. Go hiking or shopping together, then share a smoothie and ask questions.

You may feel awkward or shy about some of these topics. No problem. This book will make it easier to talk and laugh about all this.

Puberty is part of God's plan for you. It's true! God wants you to grow and learn to trust him. Yes, young girls can learn to trust God.

Did you know Mary was a teen when the angel Gabriel visited her? When she learned God chose her to be Jesus' mother, Mary could have said, "No way!" or "I'm too young." But Mary trusted God, and that helped her believe God could do amazing things through her.

Mary said yes. God chose a teenager with a heart of faith. Wow!

So for nine months, Jesus—the Author of life—grew inside this young girl. God honored Mary's body by living there. Wow, again!

God gave *your* body such respect and dignity too. This book is about your body and much more. It's about God's purpose for your life, including puberty.

So get ready for a fun adventure! Puberty comes only once, and with the changes and moods come many joys and treasures too.

> Trust in the LORD with all your heart and lean not on your own understanding; in all your ways submit to him, and he will make your paths straight.
>
> *Proverbs 3:5–6*

QUESTION 1

What does it mean to be healthy?

Have you ever been in an automobile when a tire blew? The loud KABOOM scares everyone in the car. Then the whole vehicle starts to wobble. The driver tightens her grip, slows down, and pulls over to the side of the road. As the car slows, the shaking lessens, and you hear the *plop, plop, plop* of the flattening tire. When you finally stop and get out of the car, the tire is as flat as a pancake. So much for your plans for the day.

Believe it or not, your body is designed in a similar way. Here's how.

Two of my (Dr. Walt's) very first books were *God's Design for the Highly Healthy Teen* and *10 Essentials of Happy, Healthy People*.

19

In the books, I discuss how authentic health is about a lot more than simply not being sick or trying to have the best body. I explain that health is made up of four separate parts that work together:

- Your physical health
- Your emotional/mental health
- Your relational/social health
- Your spiritual health

For example, when you have a cold (physical health), it affects your mood (your emotional health) and how you react to others (your relational health). When a girl is emotionally ill—with depression, for example—it can affect her immune system (physical health) and her relationships with her family and others (her social health).

In other words, your overall health is kind of like a car with four tires. Each tire represents an aspect of your health: your physical, emotional, relational, and spiritual health. If any one of the tires is not fully inflated, or if even one of your health wheels is not aligned correctly, it affects how the whole car rides—how well you are.

If one of your health wheels is off balance, your entire "health ride" will be bumpy. You will have to slow down to prevent a crash! And if one of your tires blows—BOOM!—your failing health stops you cold.

So even though our book is titled *The Ultimate Girls' Body Book*, it's about much more than your physical body. We'll also explain how emotional, relational, and spiritual health contributes not only to a healthier body but also to an overall healthier you.

Kate is one of the healthiest girls I (Dr. Walt) have ever known. If you met her when she was growing up and just looked at her physical body, you'd think she was not very healthy. She was born with a brain problem that keeps the muscles on her left side from working normally. As a result, they are stiff and contracted. She has a bit of a speech problem and, as a child, could only walk with braces and great difficulty. Her crossed eyes and contracted legs often caused her to stumble and fall. She was bullied frequently by kids who would mock and laugh at her.

Kate doesn't sound like the picture of health, right? Yet despite her physical disabilities, Kate's charming, genuine personality drew people to her. Most of her classmates and teachers loved her. Despite her physical challenges, Kate carried herself with class and self-respect and became highly healthy emotionally, relationally, and spiritually.

Growing up, her attitude was usually upbeat, and her infectious laugh made others smile. If she dropped something, she wouldn't get mad or frustrated; she'd just giggle. If her left hand didn't do what her brain was telling it to do, she'd say cheerfully, "That left hand has a mind all its own."

Kate loved to read and laugh out loud. She was lighthearted, even though many with similar disabilities can be heavyhearted. Not Kate. Her smile could light up the darkest room. She was also wise in choosing her friends and, as a result, was surrounded by a group of great friends who loved and helped care for her. When she needed to be in the hospital, they were always there to support her.

But most of all, Kate's deep faith in God impressed everyone around her. No one ever heard her question why God had allowed her to have such a devastating disorder. Instead, Kate would share what God was teaching her through her disabilities.

As a young woman full of kindness, gratitude, and hope, Kate was healthier than most tweens and teens I've known. Although her physical wheel was a bit out of balance, her extremely healthy emotional, social, and spiritual wheels gave her a smooth ride in life.

I had the immense pleasure of watching her grow up, and now she's a highly healthy young adult. I'm very grateful for all she's taught me. I'm even more grateful to be her dad.

So think about your health car and your four health wheels. Is there anything you can do to prevent a flat tire in your health? Or to prevent a wreck caused by a blown tire?

The answer is yes. That's the whole point of this book. There is so much *you* can do.

The first step involves prevention, which keeps things from going wrong in the first place. Like cars, people need to take good care of themselves, and they need regular checkups. During these "tune-ups," the mechanic will check the "tires" to see that they are aligned and fully inflated. If they're not, the mechanic will make the adjustments so you'll have a safe ride on the road.

I (Dr. Walt) designed a test you can take to determine if your four health wheels are healthy, or if one or more of them is flat, out of alignment, or ready to blow. You can find a link to these free evaluations for parents and tweens/teens using this QR code or the URLs included in our list of resources.

*Assess Your
Health-Teens*

The second step involves choosing to drive on safe roads that will help keep you healthy. Throughout the book, we help you learn how to drive safely when it comes to your health, and we show you what the safe roads to great health look like. As you read each question, consider how healthy you feel and what steps you need to take to get healthier if needed. We pray that this book will be a road map to becoming a healthy and godly tween and teen girl who will grow up into a healthy, godly woman.

And now, let's learn more about this exciting time of life called *puberty.*

QUESTION 2

I'm changing. What's happening to my body?

How often do you or your friends use the word *puberty*? Probably not at all. But *all* of the physical and emotional changes that you're going through are part of an ongoing conversation for most girls during the tween and teen years.

Since we are doctors—so we like medically reliable terms—we'll go with *puberty*. Here's our definition: puberty is the process that develops and changes your body physically from a girl to a woman. Here's your definition: "Wow, what's up with my body? A lot of stuff is going on!"

During puberty, your body will grow faster than at any other time in your life—well, except for when you were in your mother's womb and when you were a tiny baby. You will grow taller, you will develop hair in new places, your private parts will change, and your breasts will grow. Surely you've heard about girls getting their periods. Maybe you're wondering about *your* first period. What in the world is going on with that?

You'll also experience a roller coaster of new feelings and emotions. You can feel super confident one moment and ultrasensitive the next. In the morning, you may have it all together, only to fall apart in a single second by the first bite of your lunch. You'll have to deal with mean girls, bullying, and attraction to boys. Not to mention TV shows, movies, the Internet, videos, and video games bombarding virtually every thought you have.

We'll talk about all those things, but first let's discuss puberty, which involves three main events: the growth of your breasts, the growth of pubic hair, and your first menstrual period. Typically, the changes unfold in exactly that order and can take anywhere from two to five years. Although these changes may seem weird or even scary, they are normal, healthy, and God-designed.

Girls go through puberty at different ages and at different rates. It usually starts between the ages of eight and twelve. Over the last few decades, more girls have begun puberty before the age of eight — even down to age six or seven. And your ethnicity can make a huge difference.

If puberty starts before you're eight years old (or has not started by the time you turn twelve), you should see your doctor just to be sure everything's all right.

So what kicks off the process? Hormones do. A *gland* is a part of your body that makes the chemicals called *hormones*. The bloodstream then carries the hormones to another part of the body (like from your brain to your breasts). Puberty begins when your brain releases a bunch of these chemicals.

The hormones called *estrogen* (made primarily in your ovaries) and *human growth hormone* (HGH, made in your brain) cause most of the changes in your body during puberty. Get ready for some drama!

When these hormones reach the muscles and bones, your body's growth speeds up. If someone tells you, "You're all hands and feet," in a way they're right. During puberty, your extremities grow first, then your trunk (back, chest, and abdomen). Most girls grow fastest about six months before their first period (which is called *menarche*, but more on that later).

You'll grow taller during puberty. You'll gain weight in different places. You'll develop awe-inspiring superpowers — okay, just kidding about that last one.

Most girls will notice more body fat along the upper arms, thighs, and upper back. Your hips may grow rounder and wider, while your waist can narrow. This is all totally normal and divinely designed (that's always nice to know).

For most girls, breast growth is the first sign of puberty; estrogen causes it. Some girls will first notice hair growing in their pubic area, while a few others first notice hair growing on their arms, legs, and armpits (*axillae*). Menstrual periods usually don't come until later, typically when you're twelve or thirteen.

We know these changes can seem scary and strange to you and to other girls who go through them. But don't worry! As you learn more about what's happening, it will make sense, and you'll feel better. Trust us.

So let's begin to address the many questions that are swirling around in your mind about these amazing, God-designed changes.

> "Before I formed you in the womb I knew you, before you were born I set you apart."
>
> *Jeremiah 1:5*

> "Your Redeemer ... formed you in the womb."
>
> *Isaiah 44:24*

QUESTION 3

Why are there things about my body I just don't like?

I (Dr. Walt) was speaking to a group of fifth-grade girls at their school about their changing bodies. I looked at one of the girls, who seemed quieter than the others, and asked, "Sara, do you have any questions?" She thought for a moment and said, "How come there are some things about my body I just don't like?"

I looked around and noticed many other heads nodding. "How many of you are thinking the same thing?" Slowly, nearly every girl raised her hand. I was not surprised at all. You see, this is one of the questions we get asked most when we talk with girls about all the changes they are experiencing before and during puberty.

No matter how old you are, your body has grown, developed,

and changed over the last year. And if there is one thing we can guarantee you, even more changes are coming!

Most girls become self-conscious about their physical development during puberty. They can worry about everything—their height, weight, even the shape of their little toe. But these changes can cause even more embarrassment if your friends or parents—or even worse, boys or bullies—tease you or talk about them.

We want you to learn about and become more comfortable talking about all these changes. First, you need to consider this fact: God created you just the way you are. The Bible says God fashioned you; he formed you.

> My frame was not hidden from you when I was made in the secret place, when I was woven together in the depths of the earth. Your eyes saw my unformed body; all the days ordained for me were written in your book before one of them came to be.
>
> *Psalm 139:15–16*

God literally knit you together while you were still in your mother's womb, which the writer of the Psalm figuratively calls "the depths of the earth." In fact, the phrase "woven together" is a single word in the Hebrew that can also be translated "embroidered."

Some of you know what embroidery is: fancy and delicate stitches hand-sewn onto cloth that add beauty and value to the material. That is the word used to describe how God made *you.*

One Bible teacher wrote, "It describes the delicate embroidery of the body, the things that tie us together so that one organ supports another. The lungs need the heart, and the heart needs the lungs; the liver needs the kidneys, and the stomach needs both; all the parts are amazingly embroidered together."

In other words, God designed you. He caused your body to form and grow, like a weaver creates an art piece with yarn or string.

The Rooster Crowed

When I (Dr. Mari) got my first period, I was home with my older brother. We were watching a movie while we waited for Mom to come home. I must have taken twenty trips to the bathroom, since I didn't have a pad or any supplies to use except for toilet paper. It was a long afternoon!

When Mami (that's what we called our mom) finally came home, she was thrilled to hear the news. She hugged and kissed me and looked at me proudly, smiling, with a tender look on her face. She gave me everything I needed, like pads and some supercute undies she'd bought ahead of time to celebrate this special event. We had a great time chatting about growing up.

This beautiful mother-daughter moment was interrupted when a neighbor stopped by to borrow some sugar. Seeing all my supplies on the couch, mom's friend realized what had just happened. So at the top of her lungs, she exclaimed, "The rooster crowed!" Then, hugging me, she began to crow, "¡Qui-qui-ri-quí! ¡Qui-qui-ri-quí!"

Can you imagine?

The rooster crowed? What on earth was she talking about? The lady seemed to have lost her mind. Turns out that expression is about how a rooster crows to announce the dawn of a new day — and a new day had dawned for me. With the arrival of my first period, I was one day closer to becoming a woman.

Truth is, I still laugh every time I think about her excitement at watching me grow up. Thanks to my mom and our exuberant neighbor, I'll never forget that special day.

You are wonderfully made, which means you are special—a wonder. Your Creator has designed you to be completely unique—*one of a kind*. And he is *still* growing you—using all of these changes to shape you into the woman he has designed you to be.

> For we are God's handiwork, created in Christ Jesus to do good works, which God prepared in advance for us to do.
>
> *Ephesians 2:10*

The Greek word for "handiwork" (sometimes translated "workmanship") is *poiema* (POY-ay-mah), which means "that which is made personally." *Poiema* is also the origin of the English word *poem*, which tells us something amazing: God the Creator not only personally made you, but you are his poetry. You are his artwork. You are his masterpiece.

You are absolutely one-of-a-kind. No one else in the past or in the future has your fingerprints, your DNA pattern, your exact personality, or even the exact pattern of the veins you have on the back of your hand.

Not only does God have a blueprint just for you and your body, but he also designed a special life plan just for you. Here are two verses describing this:

> Many are the plans in a person's heart, but it is the LORD's purpose that prevails.
>
> *Proverbs 19:21*

> For it is God who works in you to will and to act in order to fulfill his good purpose.
>
> *Philippians 2:13*

God's plan for you includes using what you or others may see as imperfections. Perhaps you feel parts of your body or personality are "design flaws" — mistakes, even — but they're not. God can use all that for your benefit. He made you the way he made you for a purpose.

Do you remember Kate's story in question 1? She could have complained about her physical imperfections. Instead, she chose to see how God would use them in her life. Her disabilities allowed God to use Kate to serve in the speechwriters' office of the President of the United States. She shared the story of God's work in her life not only around the country, but also in Washington, D.C., the very center of our government.

God's plan is perfect. And God knows you. He loves you. He created you. He designed you. If you trust him, over time you will understand his design and plan for you better. This will make you more willing to follow him and even thank him for the way he made you — and even the fact that he made your little brother, who wakes you up every morning by burping your name.

You may say, "Well, it's not fair that _____." (Fill in the blank with the words "I have zits," or "I'm too short," or "My nose is too long," or any other things you simply don't like about yourself.) But if you dwell on that, aren't you really saying, "God, I don't trust your design for me. I think I know what I need better than you do."

Really?

Imagine you are God. You created the universe. You designed all of the solar systems, plants, and animals. Then you make a little girl who begins to grow into a young woman. You know why you put her together just the way she is. Everything the girl sees as a flaw, you made for a specific purpose. You know what is best for her, and you already know the end of her story. You know where she will go to school, what profession she'll choose, whom she'll marry, and what she'll accomplish.

You love that girl more than she will ever love herself. In fact, you are building an eternal home for her — so you can be together forever. And, most important, you know that at the end of her

The Hidden Masterpiece

A story is told of a young girl who was riding home from school on the subway. She'd been bullied at school that day about her looks — her acne, her tangled hair, and her hand-me-down clothes. Tears welled up in her eyes.

An older woman sat next to her and pulled out a jumble of thread that spread out several inches in each direction. There were knots everywhere, and all kinds of colors. The whole thing looked like a confused muddle of filaments going every which way.

With needle and thread, the woman began working on the mess of string. The harder she worked, the more messed up the whole thing looked. The girl laughed out loud and then covered her mouth to silence a chuckle.

"What?" the woman said, smiling. "What's so humorous about this?"

"Your sewing," the girl replied. "It just looks funny."

The woman laughed and said:

My life is but a weaving, between my Lord and me;
I cannot choose the pattern, but He works steadily.
His weaving looks confusing, as I, in foolish pride,
Forget He sees the upper, and I the underside.

The wise old woman turned the fabric over to show the girl the other side. The teen's mouth fell open as she gazed at the perfect embroidery.

The woman turned her work back over to the jumble of thread and said, "When I was your age, I would often be sad about my looks or my lot in life. I think it's true of most girls."

Years passed, and the now-grown girl reflected back on the magnificent piece of art and thought, "Only later did I learn to see myself as my Creator did. His weaving is always perfect."

life, when she meets you in heaven, she'll look back and see that your design and plan for her were perfect.

Then imagine that little girl looking in the mirror, frowning in disgust, turning red-faced in anger and pointing a finger at you, "I can't believe you made me this way. This is not fair."

If you were God, how would you feel? We know you'd still love that little girl with all your heart. But you'd want to pull her into your lap—to hug her and say, "Hang in there. Just trust in me. I don't make no junk." (Though God's grammar would be perfect.)

Part of becoming a faithful young woman who follows Jesus involves trusting that his ways are better than your ways. It might help to know that what you're going through does not surprise God.

It's perfectly okay to wonder, *God, what are you doing? What's your plan here? What are you trying to teach me?* It's honest and healthy to admit to him that you aren't comfortable with certain things. But it's wise to understand that God is God and you are not. We hope that, as you read on, this will become more and more real for you.

> "For my thoughts are not your thoughts, neither are your ways my ways," declares the LORD. "As the heavens are higher than the earth, so are my ways higher than your ways and my thoughts than your thoughts."
>
> *Isaiah 55:8–9*

> Oh yes, you shaped me first inside, then out; you formed me in my mother's womb. I thank you, High God—you're breathtaking! Body and soul, I am marvelously made! I worship in adoration—what a creation!
>
> *Psalm 139:13–15 MSG*

Hot-Cross Bonds

When pastor and author Louie Giglio looks at creation — from distant galaxies to the intricate human cell — he can't help but see the work of Jesus.

Jesus even holds our bodies together with a symbol of his never-failing love.

Pastor Giglio talks about a substance called *laminin*, which is part of a family of proteins that holds our cells together. Think of it as body glue.

Scientists who study the human cell under incredibly powerful electron microscopes have found that all laminins discovered so far are in a cross-like shape.

"How crazy is that?" Pastor Giglio says. "The stuff that holds our bodies together, that's holding the linings of your organs together, that's holding your skin on, is in the perfect shape of the cross of our Lord Jesus Christ."

God's design, love, and power are truly on display in all of creation — even in places that the human eye cannot see.

> For in him all things were created: things in heaven and on earth, visible and invisible, whether thrones or powers or rulers or authorities; all things have been created through him and for him. He is before all things, and in him all things hold together.
>
> Colossians 1:16–17

QUESTION 4

Why isn't my body changing like I expected?

I (Dr. Walt) remember having this question when I was a boy. It seemed like I was developing more slowly than all of my friends. In the ninth grade, I was a short, ninety-eight-pound weakling, with no body hair or big muscles. It seemed all of my friends were growing up faster than I was. And I *so* wanted to grow up more quickly.

We've noticed that our young patients (and their parents) sometimes worry that their growth is either too slow or progressing too quickly. If your development is ahead or behind that of your friends, you may wonder if you are normal. Chances are everything is just fine and you're right on target for your divine design.

But those girls who are on the slower end of things when it comes to their physical development tend to worry the most about this. They wonder when their breasts will grow, when they'll begin shaving hair on their legs and under their arms, or when their first period will come.

And if you're developing more quickly than other girls in your class, this can become even more painfully obvious when older boys start staring at you instead of talking to you.

It is completely normal for physical development to start at different times and move along at different rates for each girl. Once the first changes of puberty begin, it usually takes several years before all of them are complete — and on top of this, changes vary from girl to girl.

So during the teenage years, two girls who are the same age and developing normally can appear quite different from one another. You likely know some girls who look much older and more physically mature, while other friends look younger and less mature, right? But the one who starts slower will usually catch up in time.

Although your changes will be different from those of your friends, they won't be very different from your mom's (believe it or not). So if you can talk to your mom about when and how she developed, this may give you an idea of what's ahead for you.

Still, it's important to know that these days, most young girls start to grow and develop at a younger age than their moms did (about nine months earlier on average). Also, they are growing taller (about one inch taller on average) and weigh more (about ten pounds on average) than their mothers.

So how will your body change during puberty? Here are some averages:

Eight to thirteen years: Your breasts begin to grow.
Eight to fourteen years: Pubic hair begins to grow (usually after your breasts begin to grow).
Nine and a half to fourteen and a half: Your body growth speeds up and you head toward your growth spurt. *My what?* Don't worry; we'll cover that in question 5.

Nine to sixteen: You may notice hair under your arms start-ing about two years after your first pubic hairs show up. You may begin to have acne. Your sweat glands begin to produce more sweat, and it begins to smell (a.k.a. body odor or BO—more about that in question 20).

Twelve to thirteen: Your first menstrual period occurs (usu-ally after breast and pubic hair growth begins). More about that in questions 12 and 13.

Sixteen to eighteen: You are nearing your full adult height and your body shape is mature.

Remember, these are examples of *average* development. At any milestone of puberty, there is a wide range of ages.

Also, the order of events can vary from one girl to another. For example, some girls will have hair growing under their arms at the same time their leg hair is beginning to grow. Other girls could grow hair much later or much earlier.

So use these timelines as a general guide. Each of these steps will happen in the timing that God has designed for your unique system.

> Many, LORD my God, are the wonders you have done, the things you planned for us. None can compare with you; were I to speak and tell of your deeds, they would be too many to declare.
>
> *Psalm 40:5*

Your Breasts

Breast development happens in stages. The first stage, *breast budding*, starts during the earliest part of puberty. Yes, like flowers, your breasts start off as small buds.

A breast bud is simply a small raised bump behind the nipple. After breast budding, the nipple and the circle of skin around the nipple (called the *areola*) get bigger and a little darker. Then the area around the nipple and areola starts to grow into a breast.

As breasts keep growing, they may be pointy for a while before becoming rounder and fuller. A girl's breasts continue to grow throughout her teen years and even into the early twenties. Breast size is determined mostly by your heredity and your weight. So if your mom's breasts are small, it's likely that you'll have breasts of similar size. And a girl with more body fat will often have larger breasts.

Let us give you a warning: There are many companies that want you to spend money on products they claim will make your body develop faster (if you are delayed) or slower (if you are early), but the only things guaranteed to get bigger are *their* bank accounts as they take your money for products that *will not* help.

You can't do anything to make your body develop faster than God designed. Of course, you should eat a nutritious diet, stay active, and get enough sleep — we'll talk about these things later in the book. But special diets, food supplements, herbs, vitamins, or creams won't do anything to make normal puberty start sooner or happen more quickly.

Breasts are just one of many signs that you are on your way to becoming a woman. If you have questions or concerns about breasts or bras, ask your mom or a trusted adult. She knows exactly what you're going through. Also, we'll answer many of your questions about breasts in question 15.

QUESTION 5

Am I growing — or is the ceiling dropping?

Have you ever heard someone say to one of your friends, "You shot up like a weed"? Well, weeds grow much faster than regular plants and flowers, and so will you when you have your growth spurt.

Spurt is a word used to describe a short burst of activity, or something that happens in a hurry. So a *growth spurt* means your body is growing really fast.

You'll experience two kinds of growth spurts during the teen years. First, there is your *height spurt*, when you grow taller. Second, there is your *weight spurt*, when you'll gain more body fat, especially in your hips and thighs. This is God's design to make your body curvier and more feminine.

You may be surprised to learn that your height spurt is actually a series of growth spurts. You may grow a couple of inches over a few months, then grow at a normal rate for a few months, and then grow extra fast in another spurt. At some point, you will level off and stop growing once you reach your adult height.

To see if your height (also called *stature*) is normal for your age, you can use a standard stature-for-age chart like the one located at tinyurl.com/n92u7sh. In this chart, you'll notice that what's considered normal (between the 5th and 95th percentile) varies greatly. For example, on average, a twelve-year-old girl can be anywhere from fifty-four inches (about four and a half feet tall) to sixty-four inches tall (about five and a third feet tall). That's nearly a foot difference!

If you're super tall or extremely short, then your doctor should evaluate you. But if your height is in the normal range, then you may wonder how tall you will be after puberty.

A good way to predict this is to look at your parents, who gave you the *genetic code* (the unique way your individual cells are designed and arranged) that determines your height. Here is a simple formula you can use to predict how tall you *may* be when you reach your adult height (at least within three to four inches):

Note your biologic dad's height (in inches).
Subtract five inches.
To this number add your mom's height in inches.
Then divide this number by two.

Voilà! That's a guesstimate of your height when you're fully grown. However, several more accurate Internet tools can help you predict where you might end up. One tool helps you estimate your adult height based on your biological parents' adult heights. Click on this QR code or see the URLs in our resources list at the back of the book. But remember that these are simply estimates. In most cases you'll just have to wait to see how tall you become.

BMIP Calculator

During puberty, a girl can grow two to ten inches in just a few years. Your feet and hands grow first, then your facial bones, and the rest of the body follows. When your facial bones start growing before the rest of your body, your face may appear to be "long." You may feel like your nose is starting to take over your face. Your forehead will widen and your hairline will move back. But don't worry. This is all normal, and you're not going bald (even if your dad is).

Once your height spurt ends, you will not grow much taller. Toward the end of this growth spurt, the *growth plates* of your bones will fuse so that they won't grow longer. This is when you've reached your final adult height.

Although the typical girl is usually about one inch taller than most boys before puberty, women are, on average, more than five inches shorter than men. Why? Although guys generally start growing tall later than girls, their growth spurts last a lot longer. So boys catch up and eventually pass most girls.

Occasionally we'll see kids whose growth is lagging way behind. This is called *constitutional growth delay* and can cause a girl to be a slow grower or a late bloomer.

When we doctors see this, we order X-rays of the girl's bones and compare them with X-rays of what's considered average for that age. The bones of teens with constitutional growth delay look younger than what is expected for their age.

The good news is that most of these girls will have a height spurt, although a bit delayed, and continue growing and developing into womanhood. They usually catch up with their peers by the time they're young adults.

Although you may go through a stage when you feel like an ugly duckling because everything seems out of proportion, this stage will pass. You will emerge as a beautiful swan with a more mature look about your face.

In fact, you can relax, for three very good reasons:

1. You are much more aware of these changes than those around you.
2. Your trunk, or torso, will begin its growth and then your body will even out.
3. This is all part of God's perfect design for you—to transition you from a girl into a woman.

Another common worry during this stage of puberty is clumsiness, which can be embarrassing. Here's why this happens: When you grow slowly, your brain has time to adjust and learn. But when you're growing quickly, your brain has no time to catch up.

God created your brain to know where your hands and legs are at all times—even if your eyes can't see them. Don't believe it? Just close your eyes and move your fingers, hands, or feet. Your mind's eye knows exactly where they are because of a brain process with a big fancy name: *proprioception*.

Your brain works this way so it can very skillfully help guide your fingers and toes, your hands and feet, your arms and legs.

But your body can develop more quickly than your brain. So it can take your brain a little time to adapt. And while your brain is learning and catching up, you may be a bit clumsier than usual. Perhaps that's why you keep running into your dog.

But don't worry. Although this phase can be awkward and embarrassing, it will be over before you know it.

In the meantime, you can speed up your brain's learning by staying active. Exercise and active games are great ways to speed up your brain's learning and reduce clumsiness. We recommend outdoor activities and games, but for those who for safety reasons need to stay inside, games at a local gym or exercise-based video games may help.

Instead of looking down at your feet, staring at your face in the mirror, or worrying about your clumsiness, we recommend you look up to God during this time. Ask him what he's up to with you. Use this critical time in your life to take your focus off of yourself and focus on him more and more.

> The LORD makes firm the steps of the one who delights in him; though he may stumble, he will not fall, for the LORD upholds him with his hand.
>
> *Psalm 37:23–24*

Your Amazing Brain

Your brain is one of the most powerful supercomputers on the planet. The average brain weighs in at only three pounds but uses 20 percent of the oxygen you breathe and 25 percent of the calories you eat. In addition, about 20 percent of the blood flowing from the heart is pumped to the brain. Your brain is busy!

The brain needs all this constant blood flow, oxygen, and food to keep up with the heavy demands of its 100 trillion connections (*synapses*) that operate at the speed of light. The average brain has 100 billion brain cells (*neurons*) — which is amazing when you consider that the entire Milky Way galaxy is said to contain roughly 100 billion planets and stars. There's a whole universe inside your head (but don't let that give you a headache).

Your brain can handle 10 quadrillion instructions per second, which is ten times the theoretical maximum speed of the top supercomputer.

And your brain is standing by to be trained and to make you less clumsy. In fact, by practicing an action over and over, your brain can have your body do it perfectly.

If you're feeling clumsy and want to get more coordinated, try these exercises:

- Balance on one leg while moving your other leg out to the side, in front, then behind you.
- Jump in place and try to spin a perfect 180 or 360 degrees.
- Jump rope by yourself or with friends — or play hopscotch.
- Play a team sport with friends like basketball, volleyball, soccer, or field hockey.
- Stand with your feet shoulder-width apart. Lift your right knee up as you cross over your left hand and touch the outside of your right knee. Repeat by lifting your left knee and crossing over your right hand to touch it. Continue "marching" in place and touching your knee with the opposite hand.
- Run in a figure eight. Then do it backward.

QUESTION 6

Sleeping Beauty sounds boring.
Who needs sleep?

If you're the aver-
age tween or teen
girl, it's probably
safe to say you are
not getting as much
sleep as you need.
These days, more and
more young people are
staying up late and falling
asleep at school. And children arrive late at school more
often now because they oversleep.

If you're seven to twelve years old, you
need ten to eleven hours of sleep each day. Yet studies show the
average kid this age only gets eight to nine hours of sleep. That's
not enough. When you get into your teen years, you need at least
nine to ten hours of sleep each night. But most girls this age only
get six or seven hours of sleep.

This is not healthy. Your mind and body need sleep to be
in tip-top shape. If you don't get enough Zs, you may air ball

every shot at the basketball tryouts or mess up your pirouettes at your next recital—bummer. You'll have trouble getting up in the morning, concentrating, and learning at school. You may start acting like Grumpy, Dopey, or Sleepy, and you may fall asleep in class.

Also, your grades may start slipping. Kids who get the least amount of sleep are more likely to get Cs and Ds. Although study habits also play a huge role, children who sleep the most are more likely to get better grades. So getting your Zs may help you get A's and Bs.

So sleep helps your grades and it helps you stay healthy. Restful sleep reenergizes you. It allows your body and mind to recover from all of your day's activities and prepare for the next day.

Restful sleep also:

- Promotes healthy bone growth
- Helps form red blood cells that deliver oxygen to your body and brain
- Stimulates the release of human growth hormone, which helps tissues grow properly
- Strengthens your immune and nervous systems

Here's a little-known fact: The more sleep you get, the less likely you are to be overweight or obese. And if you're already overweight or obese, increasing your sleep can help you lose weight.

People who sleep fewer than seven hours a night tend to weigh more. Scientists think extra rest shuts down a gene that is tied to obesity. Less sleep also means less *leptin* (a hormone that makes you less hungry) and more *ghrelin* (a hormone that makes you hungry). People who get less sleep tend to eat a lot more, especially high-fat foods like ice cream. Hmm... perhaps Sleeping Beauty was on to something.

Yes, there may be something to the old idea of "beauty sleep." Research shows that people who don't sleep enough appear grumpier, more tired, less attractive, and unhealthier than those who are well rested. So, you see, you don't need makeup. You can just snooze your way to an ever cuter you.

Getting a good night's sleep will help you. You'll be healthier in your body and in the way you feel (your emotions). It will help

Do's and Don'ts for Healthy Zs

- Do avoid caffeine after 4:00 p.m., such as sodas, energy drinks, coffee, or chocolate. (Yes, chocolate has caffeine.)
- Do avoid exciting, violent, or scary shows, movies, or stories before bedtime. They can keep you up.
- Do stop watching TV at least thirty minutes before bed — sixty is even better. And don't use a computer or play video games for the last hour or so before bedtime. The light from the screen sends signals to your brain that it's time to wake up.
- Do keep naps short, or you might have trouble falling asleep later. You'll get the most energy from a ten- to twenty-minute "power nap."
- Don't wait until the night before to study for a big test (we sound like your parents, don't we?). Staying up all night can mess up your sleep cycle and affect how you do on the test. Plan to study ahead of time.
- Don't sleep with a pet — especially dogs — as they move around all night and can keep you from deep sleep. And if they like chewing socks and licking feet, the tickles will wake you up. This is why I (Dr. Mari) had to kick our puppy off the bed.
- Do exercise regularly, but not right before bed, which can make it harder to fall asleep. People who exercise for at least thirty minutes most days have more restful sleep than those who don't.

your relationships with your family, friends, teachers, and God. You may even become a better student and athlete.

So what are you waiting for? Go take a nap so you won't be grumpy or mean.

- Do try to go to bed and wake up around the same time each day. A *circadian clock* in your brain regulates your sleep-wake cycle. If one part of the cycle is off, it messes up the rest. Consistent bedtimes and wake-up times will help your body's clock work better. Try not to sleep in too much on the weekends, except to catch up during the occasional poor sleep week.
- Do get into bright light in the morning. It will wake you up and get you going.
- Do unwind from the day by praying, reading your Bible or a peaceful book, or journaling. Establish a regular, relaxing bedtime routine such as soaking in a warm bath and then reading or listening to soft music. This helps separate your sleep time from activities that can wake you up or stress you out.
- Do keep all computers and cell phones outside your bedroom. And turn them off at night. Keeping them on in your bedroom may keep you from having a good night's sleep, and a midnight text sent by a night-owl friend could keep you up for hours.
- Do make sure your room is cool, quiet, dark, comfortable, and free of *any* interruptions. Consider using blackout curtains, eye shades, ear plugs, "white noise," humidifiers, fans, and other devices to help you get the great night's sleep that is part of God's divine design for you.

When you lie down, your sleep will be sweet.

Proverbs 3:24

Even youths grow tired and weary, and young men stumble
and fall; but those who hope in the LORD will renew their
strength. They will soar on wings like eagles; they will run
and not grow weary, they will walk and not be faint.

Isaiah 40:30–31

QUESTION 7

Do I really need calcium for my bones?

Each year about two million broken bones (*fractures*) occur in older women because of weak bones. And many of these fractures can be prevented—especially if you take good care of your bones now, during your tween and teen years.

Calcium is a building block for strong bones. When there's not enough of it in your bloodstream, your body tries to pull calcium from your bones, which thins and weakens them—not cool. Over time, this can cause a disease called *osteoporosis*, which leads to breaks and fractures. Older people usually get this, but what you do now can keep you from getting it later.

By the time you are in your early twenties (which will be here before you know it), you'll have acquired almost 90 percent of the bone strength that you will have for the rest of your life. We doctors call this your *bone mineral density* (BMD). And from your thirties onward, no matter what you do, your BMD drops.

To have the strongest bones possible, you have to begin to take good care of them during your tween and teen years (when girls are less likely than boys to get enough calcium). Less than 10 percent of girls ages nine to seventeen get the 1,300 mg of calcium experts say you need each day. Yipes! So what can you do to get what you need?

Almost all North American girls get 300 to 400 mg of calcium each day in the foods they eat. If you add a serving of fat-free milk, soymilk, yogurt, or calcium-fortified orange juice to your breakfast, you'll get another 300 mg or so. Now you're over halfway to what you need.

Then if you add another serving of dairy (skim milk or yogurt) with a calcium-fortified whole grain cereal, you can get another 600 to 900 mg of calcium. This healthy formula will give you all the calcium you need in a day—just with a good breakfast.

We join most experts in recommending you get as much calcium as you can (if not all) from food—not pills.

If you can't get enough calcium from what you eat, your doctor or pharmacist can recommend a supplement.

Also, we can't talk about calcium without mentioning vitamin D. Your body won't absorb calcium without its BFF—vitamin D. Since it's hard to get enough vitamin D from food and potentially risky to get it from the sun, most experts currently recommend that teens take a supplement of 1,500 to 2,000 IU of vitamin D_3 daily with a meal.

Your pharmacist can help you find tasty chewable calcium and vitamin D supplements. However, when it comes to vitamin D, most multivitamins do not have what you need. Since these recommendations may change over time, be sure to discuss these suggestions with your doctor.

Sources of Calcium

This great list of calcium-rich foods comes from the CDC's Best Bones Forever website.

FOOD	PORTION	MILLIGRAMS OF CALCIUM
MILK		
Fat free	1 cup	306
Lactose reduced, fat free	1 cup	300
YOGURT		
Plain, fat free	8 ounces	452
Fruit, low fat	8 ounces	343
CHEESE		
Pasteurized Swiss	2 ounces	438
Ricotta, part skim	1/2 cup	335
Pasteurized American	2 ounces	323
Mozzarella, part skim	1.5 ounces	311
FORTIFIED FOODS		
Soy drink with added calcium	1 cup	368
Orange juice with added calcium	1 cup	300
Tofu with added calcium	1/2 cup	253
Cereal with added calcium	1 ounce	236–1043
Cereal bar with added calcium	1 bar	200
Bread with added calcium	1 slice	100

Did You Know? Fun Facts About Your Bones

Here are some fun facts about human bones from the blog *Healthy Times*:

- You have over 230 moveable and semi-moveable joints.
- Your smallest bone, the *stapes* or stirrup bone, lives in your middle ear. It transmits sound vibrations into your hearing system in the brain and measures about a third of a centimeter — that's one tiny speaker!
- Your thigh bone (called the *femur*) is stronger than concrete. It's the biggest and strongest bone in your body.
- Babies don't have kneecaps. Their kneecaps are still soft cartilage that gradually hardens into bone. This process is called *ossification*.
- At birth, you have up to 350 bones. As you grow, the number drops to 206. No, they didn't go join a percussion band. But between ages twelve and fourteen, some of your smaller bones fuse together into larger, bigger, and stronger bones.
- More than half of a grown-up's bones are located in the hands and feet.
- Your ribs move about 5 million times a year — every time you breathe.
- Did you know that humans and giraffes have the same number of bones in their necks? Seven. Giraffe neck vertebrae are just much, much longer.

Besides getting the right amount of calcium and vitamin D each day, what else can you do to have the strongest bones possible?

Stay active. Step away from the computer. Girls who spend most of their time sitting have a higher risk of osteoporosis later in life than active girls. Walking, running, jumping, dancing, and light weightlifting (for older girls only) can help strengthen and maintain healthy bones.

Avoid alcohol. Beyond all the other problems caused by alcohol, which we'll talk about in question 29, drinking also increases your risk of weak bones and fractures later in life.

Avoid tobacco. Smoking causes bad breath, stains teeth, and kills people from lung and heart disease and cancer. Smoking also weakens bones. It's just another reason to never even think about smoking.

Always remember that a nutritious diet, regular exercise, and some supplements (if needed) will go a long way toward giving you the healthiest bones possible.

> Did you not ... clothe me with skin and flesh and knit me together with bones and sinews? You gave me life and showed me kindness, and in your providence watched over my spirit.
>
> *Job 10:10–12*

QUESTION 8

Beauty. Our culture is obsessed with it. Only, most people are obsessed with the wrong kind of beauty.

In our culture, it's all about how you look on the outside. Yet, to God, your beauty begins on the inside — in your heart — and comes from that place where you were "fearfully and wonderfully made." Did you ever hear that phrase? It comes from Psalm 139.

> I praise you because I am fearfully and wonderfully made;
> your works are wonderful, I know that full well.
>
> *Psalm 139:14*

> The LORD does not look at the things people look at.
> People look at the outward appearance, but the LORD looks
> at the heart.

1 Samuel 16:7

So whether you realize it or not, you *are* a wonderful creation. That's a fact. But do you believe it? Do you feel like God's wonderful handiwork, or do you compare yourself with the supermodels on TV?

We have great news for you. Your days of rating yourself against the external beauty of photoshopped models can come to a screeching halt today. And here's why: You are, in fact, a God-designed, God-shaped, beautiful, and wonderful creation.

Regardless of how you feel or how you think you look, you are beautiful in the eyes of your Creator. God's Word says that he made you *wonderfully*. He took extreme care to craft every detail. You don't need to put on a drop of makeup or fix your hair for God to look at you and smile. He made you just the way you are, and he considers his creation—you—beautiful.

And here's more: Not only are you beautiful in God's eyes, but also your imperfections have a purpose. Did you ever think of that? Even though you are not perfect, every part of you was planned perfectly. Nothing about you is an accident. Nothing!

Your worth, value, and beauty do not come from anything outside of you. Your worth comes from having been created in the image of a good and loving God. Your beauty and value come from the love and dignity that God placed within you. It's a done deal; God made you that way.

So here you are, a young lady—beautiful in God's eyes—in the midst of a world obsessed with the wrong things. Our culture yells out lies about true beauty at every turn, from commercials to advertisements to the latest TV shows and movies. You don't have to watch for too long to see what they're selling—if you're not big-chested, tall and skinny, all made up, and willing to show some skin, you're not beautiful—at least in *their* opinion.

This message is a lie—a hurtful and destructive lie. But when the message is repeated continually, it begins to stick without you even noticing it. If you're not careful, it can become your yardstick, even your goal.

The truth is that inner beauty affects your outward appearance. Beauty that comes from the inside out reveals itself in love, joy, peace, gentleness, and kindness. It attracts others because it is true beauty.

Perhaps your grandmother or an older woman in your life can help you understand beauty in a new way. When I (Dr. Mari) was growing up, a lady in her eighties named Mary lived across the street. After her husband died, the neighborhood kids became her new family. She taught us to play card games and dominoes, and she shared with us an unlimited supply of soda and treats. Games and sweets—her house was a hit.

Mary's face was full of wrinkles, and her spine was curved. As she got older, she got shorter, and her head shook when she spoke. Although Mary's face would never end up on the cover of a beauty magazine, she radiated true beauty.

Mary loved us, and we knew it. It was her love that made her beautiful in our eyes. I loved to look at Mary, listen to her talk, and watch her play with us. She was beautiful!

Another great example was Mother Teresa. Though she was full of wrinkles in her old age, her acts of love and kindness made her absolutely beautiful. Her compassion, her deep love of God, and her servant heart inspired me (Dr. Mari) to become a doctor.

For over forty-five years, Mother Teresa ministered to the poor, sick, orphaned, and dying. She founded the Missionaries of Charity, which has grown to 610 missions in 123 countries. She even ranked first in the list of Most Widely Admired People of the 20th Century. Mother Teresa's life shows what happens when

God's love fills you and overflows onto others. Find out more about Mother Teresa in our resources list at the end of the book.

We find another wonderful example of true beauty in the Old Testament story of Esther. An orphaned girl raised by her uncle, young Esther was as beautiful on the inside as she was on the outside. She was physically pretty. But because of her genuineness and inner beauty, not simply her outer looks, "Esther won the favor of everyone who saw her" (Esther 2:15).

When an ungodly man threatened to destroy her people, Esther chose to trust God and risk everything to help them. A whole generation of Jewish men and women was saved because of her compassion, character, and courage. The beauty of what she did for others out of love surpassed her physical beauty.

Here's a different way to think about beauty:

> Your beauty should not come from outward adornment,
> such as elaborate hairstyles and the wearing of gold jewelry
> or fine clothes. Rather, it should be that of your inner self,
> the unfading beauty of a gentle and quiet spirit, which is
> of great worth in God's sight.
>
> *1 Peter 3:3–4*

This Scripture doesn't mean that you shouldn't wear jewelry or accessorize; that can be a lot of fun, and attractive. It simply emphasizes that true beauty goes much deeper and begins in your heart—where your thoughts and feelings originate.

Your thoughts and feelings lead to your actions—things you do that spread either good or bad in your surroundings. Acts of kindness, love, and respect will add to your beauty. Violence and angry outbursts will not.

Too much focus on outer beauty can lead to a poor body image, insecurity, and low self-esteem. Our culture's obsession with outer beauty contributes to all these problems and many more for today's young woman.

Beauty Around the World

It has been said that beauty is in the eye of the beholder. In various parts of the world, beauty is defined in very different ways.

- In some countries where many people have dark skin, they use whitening products to lighten it, whereas fair-skinned people in other nations, including the U.S., often flock to tanning salons to darken their skin. Go figure.

- Some Asian cultures consider a long neck beautiful. Girls as young as five years of age wear metal rings around their necks, adding more as they grow older, to give the perception of a longer and more attractive neck.

- Others believe that beauty lies in soft, unmarked skin, so they enrich their food with collagen, a protein, hoping for "flawless" skin.

- In some countries, people turn bird poop into a powder that's used as a facial mask to improve their complexion. Any takers?

- In other parts of the world, tattoos on different parts of the body indicate a person's social status.

- In yet other cultures, being heavy with bigger curves is considered most beautiful, and being skinny is frowned upon.

As you can see, outer beauty is, to a large extent, a matter of opinion — except when it comes to your Creator. To him, you are beautiful no matter where you live or what you look like. To him, you are absolutely precious — you are his pride and joy.

Yes, makeup and fashion are fun if done right at the right age. Your parents or a trusted adult can let you know what clothes are appropriate and what's the right age for you to start using makeup. But it's not good to focus primarily on pretty looks, because such beauty doesn't last, and it's not what true beauty is all about.

No matter what you do, outer looks will fade over time. Yet the beauty that comes from your heart will make you beautiful on the outside too. This kind of true beauty will last.

So your inner beauty comes from *who* you are and *whose* you are, *not* what you look like or what others say about you. Such beauty is pure, it is genuine, and it adds worth to everyone it touches. This type of loveliness — this true inner beauty — is a worthy goal for every young woman. And as you love and care for others throughout your life, you will reflect God's beauty and goodness even more.

> Charm is deceptive, and beauty is fleeting; but a woman who fears the LORD is to be praised.
>
> *Proverbs 31:30*

We talk more about beauty and the media in the next question. Meanwhile, you have a choice to make: you can let your culture define what's beautiful for you, or you can believe God's definition. Choose well — for the decision you make now will affect the rest of your life!

> Let the king be enthralled by your beauty; honor him, for he is your lord.
>
> *Psalm 45:11*

QUESTION 9

Why do I look so different from the girls I see on TV?

I (Dr. Mari) love going on media walks with my kids at the mall. We point out ads or displays in store windows and rate them as family-friendly, neutral, or an absolute disgrace. The mall gives us plenty of material for discussion, like half-naked women in displays and ads that are just plain disrespectful of girls and women. My kids now spot what's inappropriate in no time.

Take a look around the mall and study the billboards along the road. Consider the commercials on TV and online. How are girls and women portrayed in movies and reality shows?

These are the images from our culture's classroom. A bright young woman will ask herself, *What do they teach me about beauty, femininity, and sexuality?*

As you flip through the TV channels, you may wonder, *What does a skinny woman in a tiny bikini have to do with football? Why is a woman with cleavage and tight shorts selling hamburgers or cars?*

The reality is that ads often try to sell a product by misusing or exploiting something else, like a woman's body. One study suggests most people "are exposed to over 2,000 ads a day." Many of these ads *use* a woman's body to try to sell a product while stripping the models of what makes them human. Women (and even girls) are depicted as "things" and part of the merchandise rather than as people. As one article pointed out, "It's like they are 'bodies' rather than 'somebodies.' "

Sadly, in our sex-obsessed culture, "sexy" is what sells, and advertisers know it. They use a woman's sexuality to catch people's attention to try to sell more of their product. "Sexy" sells, and they make money. Jackpot! Trust us—if they discovered that squirrels riding bicycles would sell their products, they'd show that.

So how does this trend impact the models they use and the people who watch these ads? Every year, models and actresses get skinnier. Many admit they're obsessed with working out and dieting to attain a body that may look "sexy" to some but is actually quite unhealthy (more on that in question 10). Everything they do revolves around maintaining a "sexy" image. They neglect everything else to focus on their outer looks, while often feeling ugly, empty, and sad inside.

These models go to great lengths to maintain the image needed to survive in the fashion world. Some have collagen (a protein) injected to thicken their lips. Others get injections to soften wrinkles. Many others have surgeries like tummy tucks or breast enlargements. Believe it or not, some will even have ribs removed to eliminate *normal* skin lines so they will look even thinner. They go through risky operations, removing *normal* body parts, simply to look "beautiful." They starve themselves and work out for hours, becoming more and more unhealthy not only physically, but also in mind, heart, and soul.

A Fashion Faux Pas

Did you know that nobody actually looks like the models in fashion magazines? The models themselves don't even look like that in real life. Nobody does.

After photo shoots, digital retouching (known as *photoshopping*) takes place to remove natural blemishes and reshape models' bodies to make them look "sexy" and "beautiful" according to the magazine's definition of beauty.

Several models were interviewed following a photo shoot. After they'd posed for hours in front of the camera, every one of their photographs was photoshopped. Expecting to find the usual computerized touches that *create* a thinner waist and smaller hips and *remove* beauty marks, one model was shocked to find something else missing — a whole leg. An overzealous photoshopper kept thinning out her thigh until the leg vanished from sight altogether. Oops.

Don't let such lies become your standard for beauty. Such "beauty" is unattainable, unhealthy, and *not* God's plan for you. Choose to believe what God says about beauty instead — it doesn't need any touching up.

He has made everything beautiful in its time. He has also set eternity in the human heart; yet no one can fathom what God has done from beginning to end.

Ecclesiastes 3:11

Although most girls don't enter the fashion world planning to change their bodies, this becomes their reality. And the rest of the girl population grows up bombarded with these images that can become the standard for what you think *you* should look like. But those images aren't even real.

Pictures and video images of models are airbrushed, and their so-called "imperfections" (which are part of God's design for them) are removed with software programs. What they look like is completely unreal, a *visual lie.*

While the media and advertising experts try to define beauty for you, you can choose to think differently — to think wisely. You can sharpen your eyes and your mind, strengthening your heart with truth, to replace the lie that says you're not good enough or beautiful enough unless you look a certain way.

You may be asking, *How can I do this? How do I protect myself from this pressure to look like a supermodel? How do I invest in true and lasting beauty?*

The Bible sets a foundation to answer these important questions:

> Above all else, guard your heart, for everything you do flows from it.
>
> *Proverbs 4:23*

Your identity is not determined by your looks or who you are on the outside. You are the daughter of the Creator of the universe — a King who loves and accepts you as you are. After all, he made you that way, and he doesn't airbrush or photoshop anyone! As a young lady in a sex-crazed world, you must know who you are and whose you are.

As you get to know God better and experience his goodness and love, you'll begin to embrace yourself just as he made you. As you understand his plans for your life, you'll learn that his commands are there to keep you safe.

When you pursue *God's* best for your life, you will like your-self more — exactly as you are — while trusting him to transform you in those areas where *he* wants you to change. Not your cul-ture. Not your friends. Not that boy in history class who snorts when he laughs. But your God.

It is possible — even in this culture — for God's standard to become your own. It takes time and courage, and the choice to walk closely with him. It's the harder path. But it's the best and safest path. Like Jesus said:

> "Small is the gate and narrow the road that leads to life, and only a few find it."
>
> *Matthew 7:14*

To stay on this path, you need to fill your mind with God's truth to oppose the culture's lies. Part of guarding your heart and mind involves protecting your ears and your eyes. So watch what you watch.

TV shows, movies, and music affect your mind and heart, so choose well. Refuse to look at or dwell on things that are not edify-ing or good, such as sexual images or books that demean or exploit girls. Why waste your precious brain cells adding more unrealistic images to your brain? Read a good book instead, or choose a movie that will make you feel good about yourself, not worse.

Avoid magazines that make girls look sexy or older than they are. Think about those girl models. They need to be treated with respect, not used and abused. Check out our list of resources at the end of the book to find some magazines that are fun and informa-tive and that treat girls with dignity and respect. They will help you see yourself through God's eyes and live to honor him.

Invest your money, time, and energy in things that build you up and reinforce God's definition of beauty. Pursue things and people who help you fulfill your purpose in life rather than move you away from it.

It is difficult to go against the tide of our culture's emphasis on physical beauty and sexiness. But it is totally possible with God's guidance, with your parents' coaching, and with some good friends who will help you keep making wise choices.

If you've been obsessed with your looks in unhealthy ways—thinking too much about or spending too much time or money on your outer appearance—you are not alone. But today, you can choose a new way to look at yourself and others—with a deep appreciation for the gift of your body and your femininity.

The life the media is selling young people is empty and can lead to depression and eating disorders. Become a voice among your peers that upholds the dignity of all people—boys and girls, men and women. You and your friends can empower one another to become more aware of the impact of the media on your soul and heart.

Embrace your femininity as a beautiful gift to be nurtured, not exposed. Guard your heart, treat your body as the gift that it is, and move away from people (and things) who mistreat, demean, or try to exploit you.

> Do you not know that your bodies are temples of the Holy Spirit, who is in you, whom you have received from God? You are not your own; you were bought at a price. Therefore honor God with your bodies.
>
> *1 Corinthians 6:19–20*

QUESTION 10

Should I go on a diet?

A young woman wrote to me (Dr. Walt): "I think I may be over-weight. I'm thinking of trying one of the latest diet plans. Which one do you recommend?" Good question—listen in.

Incredible pressure is placed on girls to be thin. You'll hear about all sorts of ways to lose weight—a few that are healthy, but many that are unhealthy. We want you to be healthy in mind, body, soul, and spirit, and dieting is usually a very unhealthy behavior for tweens and teens. Here's why.

Going on a diet can mean making great choices about nutrition, like eating more fruit, vegetables, whole grains, fiber, and heart-healthy proteins and oils, while cutting back on fatty, fried foods, high-sugar foods, and highly processed food (so much for your new deep-fried brownie recipe).

But to many girls, going on a diet means making harmful choices, like skipping meals, eating too little, making themselves throw up, or not eating enough healthy, nutritious food. Not one of these is good.

Unfortunately, some girls turn to harmful (even dangerous) dieting to try to change their bodies and feel better about themselves. But they become less healthy and end up feeling worse.

Here are some disturbing facts about teen girls and dieting:

- About one in every two teen girls has tried dieting to change the shape of her body.
- Of teen girls at a *healthy* weight, more than one in every three try to diet anyway.
- Teens who don't feel good about themselves are more likely to diet.
- Compared with teens who don't diet, teens who do diet:
  - are more unhappy with their weight.
  - often *feel* fat even if they're at a healthy weight.
  - have lower self-esteem.
  - feel less connected to their families and schools.
  - feel less in control of their lives.

The bottom line is that if you want to achieve and maintain a healthy weight, going on a diet is usually *not* a good solution. In fact, it is often unhealthy.

First, diets rarely work. Second, over time, you are more likely to *gain* weight if you try to diet. In other words, unhealthy dieting actually causes many girls to gain weight in the long run. Why? Going without food makes your body feel deprived, and you feel sad, both of which can make you overeat later.

Dieting can make you feel hungry and preoccupied with food (thinking about it all the time). It can make you feel distracted and tired, sad and unmotivated, cold and dizzy, and deprived of foods you enjoy.

Some forms of dieting can be dangerous, such as skipping meals, using weight loss pills or laxatives, going on "crash" diets, or vomiting after eating.

As a teen, you are growing rapidly and need the right amount of nutrients to be healthy. Eliminating entire food groups or taking in too few calories when you are still developing can make you sick.

Healthy Minds and Healthy Bodies

Have you ever heard of eating disorders? This is when someone becomes so obsessed with being thin that she starts doing extreme and unhealthy things. She is afraid to gain any weight at all.

Girls with the eating disorder called *anorexia* don't eat enough. They often work out way too much, becoming way too thin. Girls with *bulimia* overeat (binge) and then they make themselves throw up (purge). Both extremes are very, very bad for their bodies and minds.

If untreated, eating disorders can harm the heart, stomach, and kidneys and can alter menstrual periods, which can also weaken a girl's bones. Girls with eating disorders can get dehydrated and have trouble sleeping. Frequent vomiting can stain their teeth permanently and lead to very bad breath.

Many of these girls have a very poor body image. They often feel fat when they're actually at a healthy weight or even too thin already. They end up not getting enough nutrition and becoming more unhealthy — even if they *look* thin or fit.

It's common for tween and teen girls to feel self-conscious, since you're changing so much. But it's not normal or healthy to feel guilty when you eat or to worry about your weight and feel bad about your body all the time. This is called having a *negative body image*. Girls (and boys) who have a negative body image often lack confidence in other areas of their lives as well.

If you worry too much about your weight or a negative body image is interfering with your life, tell an adult you trust, like a parent, teacher, coach, school counselor, youth pastor, or doctor.

Doctors don't know the exact cause of eating disorders. But we do know that society's obsession with "perfect" looks and thinness contributes to the problem. People with eating disorders are not simply obsessed with food and their weight. They are using food to deal with feelings they have about their bodies and who they are. Some of them are depressed, or they worry a lot about things they can't control. They may have family problems or very poor self-esteem, feeling like they're not good enough.

For this reason, girls (and boys) with eating disorders need professional counseling, including a doctor, a psychologist, and a dietitian. This team of experts can help a lot. But it takes time to identify and deal with the emotions that are at play behind eating disorders. It also takes time to develop a healthier relationship with food and weight, both of which are essential parts of God's design for healthy, growing girls.

You can find more information and advice at the website for the National Eating Disorders Association by using this QR code or the URL included in our list of resources.

National Eating Disorders Association

They can help you. And if the first one you ask doesn't help, ask another.

Now let's take an objective look at your weight and see if yours is healthy. It's not okay to simply guess whether your weight is normal. To objectively determine (not guess) if you're at a healthy weight, follow these steps:

> *Step 1:* Measure your height and weight accurately. Go to **http://tinyurl.com/n2x8o8j** for tips on how to do this.

For the next step, you'll need to know your height to the nearest ⅛ inch and your weight to the nearest ¼ pound. If you have trouble doing this at home, your school nurse or your doctor's medical assistant can help.

> *Step 2:* Find your Body Mass Index Percentile (BMIP). Now, follow these directions carefully. First you'll need to write down your birth date, your height (to the nearest ⅛ inch), your weight (to the nearest ¼ pound), and the date you measured your height and weight. Then, go to **http://tinyurl.com/q853fr** and enter this data. When you click on "calculate," it will come up with your individual BMIP.

BMIP Calculator

Once you know your BMIP, here's how to interpret the number:

- Below the 5th percentile: You are UNDERWEIGHT.
- Between the 5th and 74th percentile: You are at a HEALTHY WEIGHT. Hooray!
- Between the 75th and 84th percentile: You are at a NOR-MAL WEIGHT but AT RISK to become overweight. If this is your BMIP, you'll learn how to lower your risk in the next question.

- Between the 85th and 94th percentile: You are OVER-WEIGHT and AT RISK for becoming obese. If this is your BMIP, be sure to read the next question to learn how to avoid this.
- In the 95th percentile or greater: Your weight falls in the OBESE category. If this is the case, be sure to study the next question, "What can I do if I'm overweight?" There's a lot you can do to get healthier starting today.

Again, if you're between the 5th and 84th BMI percentiles, your weight is considered normal. But notice the tremendous variation in what's considered normal. For example, at age twelve, a girl is at a normal weight anywhere from 68 to 138 pounds — that means the normal weight for a twelve-year-old can vary by seventy pounds.

If you're in the 75th to 84th percentile, your weight is considered normal, but you are at risk to become overweight. I (Dr. Walt) recommend an Eight-Week Family Fitness Plan I developed for my patients in this category. You can find out more about this plan in the next question by using this QR code or the URL in our list of resources.

Eight-Week Family Fitness Plan

If you fall in the underweight, overweight, or obese category, see your doctor for a checkup. Don't put this off. Girls in each of these categories are at risk for significant health problems. Now is the time for your doctor to evaluate you and recommend some ways you can improve your health.

For girls who are at risk to become overweight or who fall in the overweight or obese categories, we've devoted the next question to you and your family. We share examples and simple tips that will help you get healthier and stay healthier — check it out.

Get Active

How many TV commercials do you watch every year? Take a guess.

The American Academy of Pediatrics (AAP) estimates that the average North American kid sees 40,000 commercials each year. That averages out to nearly 110 commercials every day. That means a lot of kids are spending a ton of time in front of the TV.

Studies show kids between eight and eighteen years old spend nearly four hours a day in front of a TV screen and another two hours on the computer. That's almost as much time as a full-time job.

Since you're only in school for around nine months a year, it's very possible that you spend more time in front of a screen than you do in a classroom.

If you want to live a healthy life and build a strong body and a strong mind, one of the best things you can do is get away from the TV and computer (yes, it can be done.). You don't have to join a sports team. Just walking the dog, helping with yard work, riding your bike, or playing outside with friends can help make you fit and strong.

If you really want to be radical, suggest to your parents that your family go without TV for a few weeks, a month, or even several months. Consider it a family fast. Believe it or not, many families who try this end up getting rid of their televisions.

When kids stop watching so much TV, they discover things they love to do. They also realize how much they were missing out on by not being physically active. They start to feel healthier and learn how to spend more quality time together as a family. Check out more great ideas on the "TV-free" websites using this QR code or the URLs included in our list of resources.

Get active, and get outside. Your body will thank you for it, and you will feel better too.

Become TV-Free

QUESTION 11

What can I do if I'm overweight?

We've talked about body image and society's obsession with outer looks and thinness. We've also discussed the importance of defining beauty through God's eyes rather than the hottest TV show or magazine cover. Although an obsession with weight, shape, and appearance is unhealthy, maintaining a healthy weight and BMIP *is* critical to your health. Thankfully, this is not something you need to achieve overnight.

The decisions you make now—about nutrition, activity, exercise, sleep, and the use of tobacco, alcohol, and drugs—will make a difference for the rest of your life. Are you willing to decide right now to live a healthy lifestyle so you'll live longer and better?

Medical studies confirm that the nutrition, exercise, and sleep habits you begin in middle school and high school are the habits you'll likely continue for life. So choosing now to eat well, exercise, and get a great night's sleep is a wise investment in your future. These are great ways to become healthy and feel better physically and mentally. Even if you're overweight now, you can regain control of your health with some simple, consistent new choices.

Do not, for a minute, believe that excess weight will disappear without you making some real changes. Most overweight and obese girls who do not make healthy changes will *not* outgrow it. If you don't start making some changes, and start soon, chances are you will be overweight or obese as an adult. You're developing habits now that may be harder to break later on. But there's a lot you and your family can do starting now.

You may be asking, *Why does this matter?* Well, if you're obese as a young girl, you have a much higher chance of developing heart disease or diabetes as early as your twenties. Worse yet, you're also more likely to die younger than your friends who have a healthy BMIP. Overall, obesity can shorten your life by somewhere between five and twenty years. Who wants that?

We're not telling you this to scare you, but to inform you of the risks of staying at an unhealthy BMIP. In every question of this book, we want to give you information that is medically reliable and biblically sound—even if the news is bad.

Why? Because in most cases, any bad news we give you can be balanced by some very good news.

Even if your weight is normal, this information can help you develop and maintain a permanent healthy lifestyle. The most common choices leading to overweight and obesity include:

1. Eating too many foods high in bad sugars (sweets or sugary drinks) and bad fats (including processed, junk, and fast foods)

2. Too much screen time (TV, computer, video games, texting, social media, etc.) and not enough active play and exercise

3. Staying up too late and getting less than nine or ten hours of sleep every night (covered in question 6)

These poor choices can lead to physical diseases (such as heart problems, high blood pressure, diabetes, arthritis, stroke, and some types of cancer), emotional problems (such as depression, anxiety, and a poor self-image), and relationship problems—all at surprisingly young ages. In fact, being overweight or obese is associated with more lasting medical and emotional problems than smoking or drinking alcohol. Yikes!

If you're an overweight or obese tween or teen, believe it or not, your body could already be building up to diseases that can harm you, even if you feel well right now. To help prevent these problems, here are some strategies to help you and your family start making better choices today.

Strategy 1: Choose healthier foods.

- Eat a wide variety of foods every day from all the food groups.
- Eat a healthy breakfast every day.
- Serve your own food, and serve it on a smaller plate. Kids who serve their own food on smaller plates eat less and feel as full as kids who eat off larger plates.
- Eat when you are hungry, and stop when you are satisfied (no, you don't have to finish all of the food on your plate—be sure to tell your mom we said this).
- Choose water or fat-free (skim) milk instead of soft drinks or juice.
- Choose foods that are high in whole grains like bran, wheat, and rye.

- When you eat out, watch your food portions. In many restaurants (especially fast food) portions are much bigger than most people need. Why not split a meal with a friend or two?
- Don't rush. Be sure to enjoy conversation with your friends or family during a meal. You'll eat more slowly, you'll eat less, and you'll fill up more quickly.
- Don't use food to make yourself feel better when you are bored, sad, or upset.
- Don't eat in front of the TV or computer.

Not all calories are healthy calories. Be aware of the amount and quality of food you eat — without obsessing over it. Learn to read food labels. Look for nutritional content. If you don't know how, you can learn by using our list of resources, or from your parents, school nurse, or a registered dietitian.

Eating foods high in protein and healthy fats helps your body and overall health. Dried fruit and nuts, bananas, avocados, string cheese, and peanut butter give you energy and are healthy choices. But foods that give you calories with little to no vitamins or minerals are known as *empty calories*. Sodas are a great example of empty calories. Sodas make you gain weight while providing no nutrition at all. So leave the soda for Yoda.

Follow this formula: 5–2–1–0.

Five: Eat five servings of fruits and vegetables every day.
Two: Two-hour screen time limit (Internet, TV, video games, phone) or less.
One: Exercise (do something active) one-half to one hour most days.
Zero: Consume zero sweetened beverages (like soda) daily.

Strategy 2: Reduce screen time and increase active time.

Physical activity is an important part of maintaining a healthy weight. It's also a great way to feel good about yourself. Spend some time every day doing physical activities you like with people you like. Start slowly, building up to the recommended 150 to 180 minutes per week—which can be, for example, thirty minutes a day, five or six days a week. The minutes you exercise each day do not have to be all at once. Ten minutes here and ten minutes there can really add up.

It's also a good idea to build up a little muscle with strength training. But don't confuse strength training with weight lifting, bodybuilding, or power lifting, which can put too much strain on young muscles, tendons, and areas of cartilage that haven't yet turned to bone (called *growth plates*). Strength training (done right) can be very helpful, and not just for athletes. Here are some benefits:

- Stronger muscles and greater fitness
- Stronger bones and joints, which means fewer injuries
- Healthier blood pressure and cholesterol levels
- A more active metabolism
- Helps you stay at a healthy weight

You can do many strength-training exercises with your own body weight (like push-ups) or by using inexpensive resistance tubing. Free weights and machine weights, used carefully and with adult supervision, are other options, but they're for older teens and adults.

Children under eight years old should not begin strength training. But as early as eight years old, strength training can become a valuable part of an overall fitness plan—as long as you use proper technique.

Strategy 3: Get a good night's sleep—every night.

Most teens need nine to ten hours of sleep a day—and most get only six to seven hours. Not getting enough sleep can make it hard to pay attention at school. That means lower grades. And it can make you cranky and emotional, affecting your relationships with your family, friends, and teachers. Ever see cartoons of Donald Duck? He's got a pretty short fuse, right? Not getting enough sleep makes you a bit like that—nap so you won't quack.

And get this: not getting enough sleep can make you gain weight because of two hormones called *ghrelin* and *leptin*. Ghrelin causes you to gain weight, while leptin helps you lose weight. The less sleep you get, the more weight-gaining ghrelin and the less weight-losing leptin you produce. Who wants that?

If you get enough sleep each night, exercise most days, and eat nutritious foods, you're much more likely to reach and maintain a healthy weight. (See the answer to question 6.)

So, do you think you're making wise decisions in these areas? Do you want to know for sure? I (Dr. Walt) developed a simple quiz you can take to test your nutrition and exercise habits. You can find the SuperSized Kids Test at www.supersizedkids.com /resources/quiz/index.

After you finish the quiz, you'll receive three grades in three areas: activity, nutrition, and family BMI. Completing this questionnaire will give you an instant snapshot of your risk status. If you don't make straight A's, don't be alarmed. Very, very few teens do.

To help you improve your health grade, I (Dr. Walt) joined with nutrition expert Cheryl Flynt, RD, MPH, and the experts at Florida Hospital in Orlando to develop and test an eight-week family fitness program that you and your family can use to get healthier. The program is easy and fun and designed for everyone in your family (except babies). In many families, the tween or teen can become the organizer and encourager for her mom, dad, and siblings. You can get the Eight-Week Family Fitness Plan for free using this QR code or the URL included in our list of resources.

Eight-Week Family Fitness Plan

Show your ideas to your parents. Schedule a family meeting to discuss any challenges you identified when you took the quiz on exercise and nutrition. Talk about possible actions you could take as a family. See if your siblings and parents have any other ideas and find out what you'd all be willing to try.

Once you have a plan, it's time to get started. Remember, small changes can result in big benefits. The simple steps in the eight-week plan will work. In fact, you can meet other families with kids your age (on the SuperSized Kids website) who have used the plan with success. Go to tinyurl.com/bklelw4 to check it out.

Don't give up. At the end of the eight weeks, retake the Super-Sized test to see how much you've improved. If your family enjoys the first eight weeks, a second eight-week plan that's a bit more advanced is available at http://tinyurl.com/bxabe94.

By the way, the eight-week plan can be done once a week for eight weeks, or twice a month for four months, or once a month over eight to ten months. How quickly or slowly you do it doesn't matter. The main thing is to get started and to finish together.

One last word of encouragement. Adults who are overweight or obese have only one way to get their BMIP into a healthy range. They must lose weight. But as a tween or teen, you're getting ready to enter into a growth spurt. Growing in height means that, for many overweight girls, there may be no need for weight loss at all. As your height increases, your BMIP may just slowly drop into the normal range.

That's why we encourage girls to begin developing healthy habits—to become fitter and healthier—as opposed to dieting or trying to lose weight. Some girls may have some weight to lose—but this should only be done under the direction of your doctor.

Becoming fitter and healthier takes discipline, work, and time. But think of it like this: If you put a little money in a savings account each week, the interest builds slowly, barely noticeable at first. But as time goes on, the interest grows faster and faster.

It's the same way with your health. Good habits now build interest for a long and healthy life. Even if you don't recognize it

The Lopez Family — Daughter Age 11, Son Age 13

Angel Lopez is a single father with two children, Aimee, age eleven, and Angel III, age thirteen. He wanted to rescue his children from the obesity threat and motivate them to take better care of their health.

With a family weight of 549 pounds, Angel looked for something that would help them make lasting changes in their eating and activity habits. Angel III realized this would not be so easy for him. He loved to watch TV and play video games — both of which are linked to weight gain.

Aimee and her dad decided they could start by going for walks together before preparing dinner. They decided to watch less TV and never eat in front of the TV. When they went out to eat, they tried to choose healthier food. And Aimee and her dad began working out together at a local fitness center.

Other changes that helped them succeed included:

- Spinning classes at the gym
- Adding "screen-free" nights
- Eating more whole grains and protein
- Spending more time playing outside than looking at a screen

The results after eight weeks were remarkable. The Lopez family lost forty-two pounds.

now, as you get older, you'll be thankful for the choices you made. To a large extent, you control how healthy you will be. God gave you an amazing body. It's your job to feed it right and make sure it gets enough exercise and sleep.

> Long life to you! Good health to you and your household!
> And good health to all that is yours!

1 Samuel 25:6

QUESTION 12

Some of my friends are having periods; others aren't. What's up with that?

So you've arrived at the question that part of you has wanted to read — and part of you has wanted to avoid. But there's no way around it. Menstrual periods (or *menses*, what most girls call periods) are a normal part of every girl's development.

Perhaps you've already had periods. If not, your first one may be just around the corner, or you may still have a few more years to wait. The first period comes at different ages for different girls. This is normal. But here are some guidelines to help you estimate when your first period will arrive, though not to the day.

Most girls begin to develop *secondary sexual characteristics* when they're eight or nine. These include growing breasts and body hair, among others. In general, your first period will come about two years after your breasts begin to grow. This is usually between the ages of ten and sixteen.

About six months or so before your first period, you might notice more clear discharge on your panties. This is very common. In general, there's no need to worry about this *vaginal discharge* unless it has a strong odor or causes irritation, itchiness, or other symptoms. See your doctor if you're not sure.

When your first period arrives, you've reached the stage of puberty called *menarche*, and your body's clock has begun a cycle that will repeat itself about every twenty to forty days. A *menstrual cycle* is the length of time (in days) between one period and the next. So if you got your period on January 1 and the next one started February 1, that cycle lasted thirty-one days.

Although you may have heard that the typical menstrual cycle lasts twenty-eight days, that figure is just an average. This means that, for most girls, the time between one period and the next *averages* twenty-eight days, but a completely normal menstrual cycle can be as short as twenty days or as long as forty days. And the cycle length can be different from cycle to cycle, especially in puberty. All this is very normal.

You may wonder how long the typical period lasts. Here again, this varies a lot, but most girls will have about three to five days of bleeding, although it can last up to ten to twelve days.

In the two years after your very first period, your cycles will vary a lot (how long they last, how many days you bleed, and how much you bleed). Your cycles can be quite irregular. You may have a period with light bleeding or spotting that lasts a week, then no period for two or three months. Then you get a longer one, say, for about ten days, with heavy bleeding, then you skip another month and have a shorter one, and so on. You may feel cramps with some periods. Other times, you may feel nothing at all. Every part of your cycle can vary like crazy.

Then, after that first year or two of somewhat erratic peri-ods, your menstrual cycle becomes more consistent and your periods become more predictable. Yes, this day will come. Just be patient.

Let us caution you about something that has become popular. Because of the availability of birth control pills (called *the pill*), girls and their moms will sometimes ask doctors for this medication to "regulate" a girl's cycle. Have you heard of this?

In general, this is not a good idea and rarely needed. The pill is a combination of powerful hormones (estrogen and progestin) that can cause many serious side effects. Your periods will improve over time on their own without the pill. So why risk the side effects (like nausea, headaches, depression, and blood clots) that can arise from taking extra hormones that you don't really need? Learning about your cycles and the normal monthly changes in your body will help a lot.

Since your initial periods will likely be unpredictable, you need to be prepared. So always carry one or two sanitary pads with you. There are a few different types from which to choose.

One type is an external pad that attaches to your panties just outside of your vagina. A second option is a "plug-in" pad, known as a *tampon*. Either type can keep the fluids that come with each period from getting on your clothing.

You can keep sanitary pads and extra panties in your purse, backpack, and/or locker. That way when a period comes unexpectedly, you'll be ready.

Even so, your period may still catch you by surprise at times. If it does, don't worry. You can fold toilet paper into a rectangle and use that as a sanitary napkin until you can get a pad. Usually other girls or women — a friend, teacher, school nurse, coach, or office staff — will have some extra pads. It's perfectly okay to ask for one. If someone helps you, you can bet that this has likely happened to her too.

When it comes to choosing between a pad and a tampon, talk to your mom or a trusted adult. She will help you get the right products for you. Most girls use a sanitary liner (a pad) rather

Premenstrual Blues

Periods are a part of life for growing girls. Period. You're either on your period, getting over your period, or about to start your period, and each one of these stages of your monthly cycle is caused by changes in hormone levels. You had no idea that being a girl had so much to do with science, did you?

As hormone levels go up and down, so does your mood. Did you ever hear about *premenstrual syndrome*, or *PMS*? This simply describes how you may feel right before a period. You may feel super moody, more tired, or just plain blah. You may feel down and unmotivated, irritable or cranky. PMS is common and happens to all women to some extent, and you can do a lot to keep it under control.

To prevent or decrease PMS symptoms, be sure to

- eat well,
- exercise, and
- get enough rest.

If you do this consistently, studies show that your whole monthly cycle will be much better. You will feel less crampy and less achy, and your moods will be more stable. Why not give it a try?

Stay active right before and during your period. This is extremely helpful. Also, healthy eating makes a huge difference. Girls with high-fat, high-carb diets, especially right before their period, will have lower "lows" than those who eat more fruits, vegetables, and fiber-rich foods.

If you have extreme PMS symptoms every month, you may have moved from PMS to what is called *premenstrual dysphoric disorder* (PMDD), where the symptoms of PMS begin to really affect with your life. If you consistently have what seems to be severe PMS month after month, see your doctor to get help.

than tampons. Most doctors recommend external pads because they are safer, especially for nighttime use.

Some external pads come with wings, which means they extend to the sides, not just front and back. They protect your underwear better, especially on heavy flow days. You can find brands that are thicker and more absorbent — they're for heavier periods. You can use thinner pads on light flow days. You may want to have both types around, since your flow can be heavier the first few days of each period and then lighten up.

Rachel's Timely Period

Menstrual cramps have been around since Adam and Eve. We know this because the Bible talks about periods in Genesis, where we read a story about Rachel trying to hide some items she had stolen from her father. She placed the items under her camel's saddle and sat on them. And then:

> Rachel said to her father, "Don't be angry, my lord, that I cannot stand up in your presence; I'm having my period." So he searched but could not find the household gods.
>
> Genesis 31:35

She got away with using her period as an excuse and a distraction — sneaky Rachel.

It could be tempting to use your period as an excuse to sit around and do nothing for days, but there's no need for that. Nowadays, there's a lot you can do to reduce your cramps and continue to enjoy life during this time of the month.

Still, you may feel moody or irritable, and your breasts may feel swollen. You may feel bloated and get cramps or soreness

A tampon is an absorbent cotton "plug" that's inserted into the vagina with a plastic or cardboard applicator. Your mom, an older sister, a trusted woman, or even your doctor's nurse can show you how to safely insert a tampon into your vagina. Tampons are particularly useful during athletic activities. They can even be worn while swimming. But we want to stress that tampons are for *daytime* use only.

If you choose to use a tampon, you've got to remember to change it every few hours. Why? You want to avoid the risk of

over the uterus and pubic area. Sometimes your lower back or upper thighs may feel uncomfortable. This is common, typically mild, and it doesn't have to interfere much with your life.

Warm baths can help your tummy feel better. A warm towel or heating pad (on a low setting) placed over the lower abdomen will also help. You can also take an over-the-counter medication like acetaminophen, ibuprofen, or naproxen. This can be extremely helpful, and when taken as directed, it is usually safe. Ask your doctor or pharmacist which medication is right for you. To help reduce bloating, stay away from salty foods and caffeine and drink more water.

If these simple measures don't control the cramping and mild discomfort that come with normal periods, or if you have moderate or severe symptoms, make an appointment with your doctor.

But don't be like Rachel — you'll feel a lot better if you get off your camel and move.

a serious infection known as *toxic shock syndrome* (TSS). TSS can be horrible. It can make you seriously ill, or rarely, it can even be fatal. Because of this, tampons are *not* a good option for someone who is forgetful. It could be very dangerous if you forget that you're wearing a tampon and leave it inside for too long. That's another reason we never recommend tampons for nighttime use.

Vitamins and Minerals for PMS

Although most girls don't need to take anything at all for PMS, some vitamins or minerals may help those girls who have more symptoms right before their periods. The doctors of pharmacy at the Natural Medicines Comprehensive Database recommend:

- Calcium: Taking 1,000 to 1,200 mg daily seems to lessen water retention, pain, and "the blues" that can come with PMS. You can read more about calcium in question 7.
- Pyridoxine (vitamin B_6): Taking 50 to 100 mg daily can improve PMS-related breast soreness and gloom.

Before you try any natural medicine (herb, vitamin, or supplement), be sure to discuss it with your physician or pharmacist. Even though these medicines are natural, they can still cause unexpected symptoms. So don't take them on your own and never take more than your doctor recommends.

The good news is that you can continue to play sports and be as active as you want even while on your period. You can go running or biking or practice almost any sport you like. You may want to use tampons for activities such as swimming or gymnastics.

Staying active during your period will minimize cramping and help you feel better, so keep moving and eat healthy foods. Remember to change your pad often (every three to four hours) and you'll be just fine.

Occasionally, a problem may present itself through a change in your normal periods. See your doctor if:

1. You have persistent bleeding between periods.
2. There is a sudden change in the normal pattern of your periods.
3. You soak more than seven or eight pads per day for longer than a week to ten days.
4. You develop severe tummy pain at any time.

Thankfully, these problems are not very common and most periods are mild and easy to manage.

Well, you did it! You got through this awkward section. We know periods are a little weird to talk about at first, but they are a *normal* part of becoming and being a woman. It's okay to feel a bit embarrassed.

God made your body this way—periods and all—for a reason. We'll talk more about that in the next question because we know you're wondering: *Why do I have to have periods in the first place? And why do periods have to come every month?*

Keep reading. Everything is about to make sense.

QUESTION 13

How do periods work, anyway?

One of my (Dr. Mari's) friends got her very first period on the day of her fourteenth birthday. She was the last of her friends to get her period. She had invited her friends over that night for a pajama party to celebrate her birthday. Here's what she says happened next:

> That day, I came home from school to get ready for the slumber party, went up to the bathroom, and discovered that I had "become a woman." My mom had already supplied me with the "necessities," so I quickly took care of it.
>
> That evening when my friends and I were all in the bathroom getting ready for bed, the discussion turned to our periods.
>
> When my friends discovered that I had mine, one asked, "How long have you had it?"

I said, "Awhile" (technically not a lie), and the look on her face was priceless.

Thereafter, I always felt like my period was God's birthday present to me. That made all of the unpleasantness that goes along with it so much easier to bear.

Although your first period may not come on your birthday, it is still a wonderful gift. Why?

You have hormones (with names like *FSH*, *LH*, *estrogen*, and *progesterone*) that rise and fall in predictable ways throughout your monthly cycle for a specific purpose. Their ups and downs are preparing your body for something special. Your periods have a lot to do with another gift you may receive someday. It is the gift of motherhood, one of the most amazing experiences a woman can have.

Here's how it's all related: From birth, girls have *ovaries*, *fallopian tubes*, and a *uterus*. Your two ovaries are oval-shaped, about the size of small pecans, and sit on either side of your *uterus* (womb). They are located in the very lowest part of your tummy, called the *pelvis*. When you are born, your ovaries each contain thousands of eggs, also called *ova*. Each egg (or *ovum*) is microscopic—smaller than the period at the end of this sentence.

Your two fallopian tubes are long and as thin as a piece of spaghetti. Each fallopian tube stretches from an ovary to the uterus, which is a pear-shaped organ that sits right in the middle of and at the very bottom of the pelvis.

The muscles in a woman's uterus are incredible—they can slowly stretch to the size of a basketball and hold a fully grown baby. Ever hear of Elastigirl? Your womb muscles are a bit like that—stretchy and strong. So you do have some superpowers after all.

According to *Guinness World Records*, the largest baby ever born (and, thus, held inside the mother's uterus) was twenty-three pounds and twelve ounces. That's the average size of an eighteen-month-old child! After all that stretching for nine months, the strong muscles of the uterus are able to begin to contract (we call that *labor*) and then push the child out when it's time for the baby to be born. Amazing!

As you enter puberty, your pituitary gland releases strong hormones (FSH and LH). These two hormones get your ovaries to make estrogen and progesterone, which cause many of the physical and emotional changes we've been talking about, including your menstrual cycles.

About once a month, a tiny egg (ovum) will be launched from one of your ovaries — a process called *ovulation* — right into the abdominal cavity. The fallopian tube is way cool. Its mouth, which is near the ovary, has amazing finger-like pods that are designed to draw the egg inside. They stretch out and then tighten — just as your fingers do when you open your hand and then make a fist. Once a finger touches the egg, all of the fingers contract and push the egg into the fallopian tube.

Once the egg is inside, the fallopian tube contracts rhythmically to push the egg toward the inside of the uterus. You can find absolutely amazing video of this on the Internet using the URL in our list of resources.

Anyway, in the days before you ovulate, estrogen will stimulate your uterus to build up its lining with extra blood and tissue, making the walls of your uterus (the *endometrium*) thick and lush. This prepares your uterus for a possible pregnancy each month. Why?

If you've already begun to have periods (or if you're just about to have your first period) and you have sexual intercourse with a male, you can get pregnant. Did you know that? Yes, as long as you're having periods, you can get pregnant if you have sex.

Let's say that again. Even while in middle school, you can get pregnant if you have sex, even if your period doesn't show up every month. (If you don't know much about sex, this would be a good time to ask your mom or trusted adult about it.)

So how does this happen? If a woman's egg joins up with a man's sperm cell, at that instant, the egg and sperm cells miraculously combine to create another human being—a new life. Once *fertilization* takes place, a brand-new, unique human being exists.

Then the newly formed human will travel down the fallopian tube to your uterus and attach, or implant, to the cushiony wall of your uterus. There, it will continue to develop as your unborn baby. Wow! By attaching to the lining of your uterus, he or she begins to grow in the safety of his or her new home. A woman's womb is the safest place on earth for God's miracle of new life.

So how is all this related to your periods? Here's how:

If your egg is released and not fertilized by a hopeful sperm—which is the case during most monthly cycles—then your body recognizes that you are *not* pregnant. Since there's no baby growing in your womb that month, those tissues that thickened within the uterus are not needed. So guess what happens? The uterus begins to contract and the excess lining (tissue and blood) leaves through the opening of the uterus (the *cervix*), into your vagina, and out of your body.

That's when your period comes. All of this blood and tissue is known as *menses*. After your period, the lining of the womb gets thin again. Then the whole cycle begins all over again, reminding girls and women that God made our bodies with a unique purpose.

This cycle happens almost every month for several decades (except, of course, when you're pregnant) until you reach the stage in life called *menopause*, when your periods stop. On average, you can wave periods goodbye around age fifty. Your periods won't last forever.

This is the science behind your menstrual period. But there are also spiritual realities involving your period that are just as important to recognize. As you begin to understand the awesome privilege of having a female body, we believe you will begin to see your periods as the gifts that they are.

Every period can remind you that God entrusted you with a gift and a responsibility. Everything that is unique about the female body, even having breasts that can nurture an infant with

Blot the Spot

Have you ever heard of "spotting"? This is when you see menstrual-like fluid during a time of the month when you're not having a period. It can look like your period is starting, but it never does. You simply "spot" for a day or two.

These are good days to wear panty liners to keep your underwear from getting stained. Such spotting is especially likely during those first two years of irregular periods. However, after that time, recurrent or painful spotting can signal a problem, such as an infection or a lesion on the cervix. If this type of spotting is an issue, see your doctor to figure out why.

milk, revolves around the possibility of the divinely designed gift of motherhood within marriage.

We've covered a lot of ground, and it all started by talking about your periods. Your monthly cycles are a great reminder of God's plan for you as a girl and as a woman who may one day be someone's mom—in God's perfect time.

So, with each period, when you are tempted to complain about the messiness or cramps, let your period remind you of the gift and responsibility that God has entrusted to you. You can even use any discomfort or messiness as an opportunity to pray.

Pray that God will help you honor him with your soul, your body, and your purity. Pray that he will help you see yourself through his eyes—every part of you. Even your periods, cramps, and moods.

What an amazing gift your body is—it's God's masterpiece. This whole process is an awesome part of God's creation.

QUESTION 14

What's that on my underwear?

I (Dr. Mari) have an embarrassing story to share with you. Years ago, I had a sleepover at my neighbor's house. The next morning we went to the beach. I was eleven years old, smack in the middle of puberty. My friend's sister was eight and hadn't started developing quite yet.

I went to the bathroom to change into my bathing suit and left my underwear on the floor. When we returned after hours of snorkeling, my friend's sister found my underwear. With a curious look on her face, she dangled my undies in front of me and asked, "What's *that* on your underwear?"

I was so terribly embarrassed. I wanted the earth to swallow me up and take me to the Land of Oz or somewhere far, far away. Thankfully, no one else was around for this awkward moment.

If I could go back in time, my answer about the normal discharge stain on my underwear would have been matter-of-fact and blush-free. The fact is that all girls see normal mucus appear on their underwear beginning around age nine or ten. About six months to a year before your first period, you may begin to see and feel mucus coming from your vagina. This is perfectly normal — God made you this way.

As all the hormone changes affect your breasts, hair, skin, brain, and moods, they also lead to fluids that end up on your underwear. What's on your undies is completely normal and God-designed.

So what exactly is this vaginal discharge? It is part of how your female reproductive organs stay clean and healthy. Your vagina and cervix (the lowest part of your womb) form fluids and mucus that carry away dead skin cells and bacteria. This can help prevent infections in the womb. Your discharge is a little bit like earwax, which keeps your ears clean. We know — double *yikes*.

You may wonder if normal discharge is stinky or what it's supposed to look like. Normal discharge can be sticky, stretchy, slippery, gooey, or tacky, and it can be clear, transparent, or a milky white shade. Although it has a natural scent, it's not a bad smell, and you'll get used to what's normal for you.

You may notice a strong odor if you're sweaty, as during sports, but washing with soap and water will remove that smell. If an unpleasant odor persists despite washing, get that checked by your doctor.

Normal discharge shouldn't itch, burn, sting, or hurt, but infections can be quite bothersome. If you become infected with a type of germ called *yeast*, it can be very itchy. These germs can overgrow in moist areas that don't "breathe" well, like under your breasts or inside your vagina. Vaginal yeast infections cause a cottage cheese–like discharge.

If you become infected with a type of germ called *bacteria*, your discharge may be frothy and yellow or green. The discharge may also burn, itch, or just feel uncomfortable. In either case, it's worth going to your doctor to check it out.

You may wonder what's the "right" way to wash the vaginal area. Soap and water is all you need. Your normal vaginal mucus takes care of cleaning the vagina itself—there's no need to help it along.

Have you heard of *douching*? This is *not* the right way to wash your vagina. Douche is a French word that means to wash or soak. Douches are mixtures of water and baking soda, vinegar, iodine, and other products that are squirted into the vagina to "clean" it. Yet most doctors and medical organizations recommend *not* doing this. It is unnecessary and can lead to infections being jetted right up inside you. So don't douche!

Observe the normal changes in your mucus throughout the month to get to know your body better. You can even identify when you're ovulating (when an egg is released from your ovary) by observing the day-to-day changes in your mucus closely. When it gets clear, stretchy, and slippery, it's egg time. This is the fertile time of the month. If a girl has sex with a boy when she's ovulating, she can get pregnant.

The next menstrual period will usually occur about two weeks after the egg is released—no matter how irregular your cycle. As you get to know your cycles, you can learn what to expect in terms of moods, breast tenderness, and other physical and emotional symptoms that may come each month.

Itch, Itch, Go Away

PREVENTING SKIN YEAST INFECTIONS

To help keep the skin around your vagina from getting sweaty, itchy, or infected with yeast:

- Wear cotton underwear, and avoid tight-fitting undies and pants. The goal is to keep those parts dry. Moisture will make yeast germs overgrow.
- If you're an athlete or dancer, bring extra underwear to practice and games.
- After a workout, wash and dry yourself and change into dry undies. You can sprinkle athletic powder in this area to help keep it dry.
- Avoid staying in a wet bathing suit too long.
- Avoid *scented* feminine pads or tampons, sprays, soaps, powder, and lotions. They can irritate your skin and contribute to infections.
- Bottom line: let your private parts breathe and keep them dry.

PREVENTING VAGINAL YEAST INFECTIONS

To prevent yeast infections inside the vagina (especially if you get them often):

- Eat a balanced diet rich in fruits, vegetables, whole grains, and nonfat dairy products.
- Some women think that eating foods with *Lactobacillus* organisms, such as yogurt or acidophilus milk, will prevent yeast infections. There's no medical evidence for this, but these foods can be part of a healthy diet.
- Ask your doctor or pharmacist about taking probiotics. These friendly bacteria can keep the harmful yeast germs under control.

- If you're getting yeast infections that are frequent or tough to treat, your doctor may need to check your sugar levels to rule out diabetes.

PREVENTING URINARY TRACT INFECTIONS

- In girls and women, the *urethra* (the tiny tube that carries urine from your bladder to the outside) is very short.
- Bacteria from your skin can travel up the short urethra and cause an infection in your bladder, a urinary tract infection (UTI). UTIs can hurt and cause burning when you pee. Ouch.
- To help prevent UTIs, wipe carefully after having a bowel movement. Always wipe front-to-back. After pooping, wiping from *back to front* can spread a troop of poop germs to the skin near the urethra — not a good move! Front-to-back wiping ensures that stinky troop of germs will stay far from your urethra and vagina. Hooray!

TREATING VAGINAL YEAST INFECTIONS

- If you develop the itchy, cottage-cheesy vaginal discharge that is so typical of vaginal yeast infections, you can buy an over-the-counter vaginal yeast treatment like *miconazole* to treat it.
- Just follow the instructions on the container.
- See your doctor if the infection gets worse or lasts more than a few days.

QUESTION 15

My breasts aren't growing. What's wrong with me?

By now you probably know exactly what we're going to say: Each girl develops at a different rate. And if your breasts aren't growing yet, they will begin to grow exactly at the time God intended—at the right time for *you*.

Sometime between the ages of eight and ten, you will notice two small, firm bumps under your nipples. You learned in question 4 that these bumps are known as *breast buds*. Initially, they may be a little sore, but that won't last very long.

One bud may emerge before the other, so don't be alarmed if things look a bit unequal at first. For most girls, one breast is a little bigger than the other. But you can always ask your doctor if you're not sure what's normal for you.

The beginning of breast development is called *thelarche*. It can begin slightly earlier for some girls or a bit later for others. Some girls seem to grow breasts overnight while their friends wonder, *Will my breasts ever grow?* It's different for each girl because God creates each of you uniquely.

During this part of puberty, some girls wonder if they can do anything to make their breasts grow faster or bigger. Despite what advertisements and magazines say, there is no magic cream, pill, or exercise that can speed up the process or make your breasts larger than they are designed to be.

Whether your breasts are already growing or just starting to "bud," you may wonder when to start wearing a bra. I (Dr. Mari) recently overheard some seven-year-olds talking about bras. They were surprised that a girl in fourth grade was already wearing a training bra. Then one turned and asked, "When will I need to start wearing one?"

I was amazed that, in second grade, girls talk about training bras. I explained that girls' bodies develop at different rates and that she likely still has a few more years to go. Some girls begin wearing a bra in late elementary school, whereas others start in middle school. Both are perfectly normal.

Rather than wearing a bra early on, some girls prefer a light undershirt. Talk to your mom or a trusted adult about what you prefer and do what's most comfortable for you. One thing we've noticed is that some girls are thrilled to be old enough to start wearing a bra, whereas others are not at all excited. These are both common reactions, and you'll soon get used to the whole thing. Do what makes you feel most at ease during this time of change.

Bras can be very helpful. They help support your growing breasts, especially during exercise, and they also help you dress more modestly as your breasts grow larger.

When your breasts begin to grow, you can wear a training bra, which is a lightweight, pullover type of bra for growing girls.

A lot of girls prefer to start off with a camisole, which is a comfy and lightweight tank top.

Breasts come in all sizes, and they change over time. But whether your breasts are like buds, fried eggs, growing apples, or full-grown watermelons, all girls eventually need a few good bras. Songs have been written (and sung brilliantly) about the importance of a comfy "over-the-shoulder-boulder-holder." So be sure to have some fun with this.

Shopping for Your First Bra

Once your breasts begin to grow, it's time to shop. You get to handpick your first few bras. Plan a fun day out with your mom, aunt, or older sister and go shop for bras together. Let her help you find the right style and, more important, the right size. You want a bra that's comfortable and doesn't slide all over the place or feel tight.

It can take a little while to get used to wearing that first bra — they can be tricky. They can be difficult to fasten and adjust. They may dig in, ride up, slide off your shoulders, or peek out of your clothing, especially if you don't have just the right bra for your body shape and activity.

A bra can even snap open right as you spike a volleyball with all your might — WHAM! POP! Uh-oh! Yes, that happened to me (Dr. Mari) in high school.

Several department stores offer free bra fittings. We know what you're probably thinking: *Fitted? I need to get fitted? What is this — the prom?* Don't worry. No need to fret over that first fitting. (You can do measurements at home first. While at home, have your mom or sister or trusted adult measure your chest size all the way around the fullest part. Then measure around your chest under your breasts. Write down these two numbers and

Have you noticed the numbers and letters on bras, like 28A, 28AA, 32B, or 36C? In bra language, the *number* refers to your chest size (the total inches at the widest point around your chest) when measured with a measuring tape. The *letter* refers to cup size (the measurement of the breast itself), as in the triangular section that covers your breast like a bikini top.

As your breasts grow larger, your cup size increases. You may start out with an A or AA cup. Lots of girls may start with a

bring them with you.) Then choose a department store to go try on some bras.

Most stores have a clerk who is trained to help fit girls for their first bra. She can help you figure out your cup size (the letter) and can teach you how to adjust the straps. Although you may feel awkward going there and asking for help, the ladies in the bra section do this all the time. It will really help to have a woman trained to fit bras measure you and suggest the best bra size for you. Fittings at these stores are done discreetly in a fitting room, so it will be private and not embarrassing.

One of our reviewers, who works at one of these stores, wrote:

> I see young girls coming in for their first bra fitting all the time. They are usually really nervous and shy and maybe feel a little awkward about getting a fitting, but it is very important that they do come in to some professional place for that fitting ... [and] start off with the right bra from the beginning.

It's perfectly normal to feel a bit embarrassed when bra shopping for the first time, but don't worry. All girls and women go through this. We're all in this together.

sports bra, which provides support for running, jumping, and more active days. Not all bras are alike, so you'll have to try some on or get fitted.

Once you know your size, walk around and pick out your favorite designs. If you're looking to smooth out your growing breasts and nipples, a training bra will do the trick. If you want more support for your active lifestyle, a sports bra is the way to go. For all other needs, a regular bra will suffice.

Your new bra should feel comfortable. If it feels tight, choose a different style or a larger size. Adjust the straps if needed; that can really help when a bra wants to ride up and dig in. Along the way, ask questions about bra styles and don't forget to laugh. You'll likely remember this day for a very long time.

Before we finish this question, let us give you a warning. There's one thing you may experience that can feel awkward: While in school or playing sports, you may be sent to the locker room to change into your physical education (PE) or sports clothes. You will notice that some girls change in front of each other, whereas others prefer the privacy of a bathroom stall. Many girls feel uncomfortable when thrown into the chaos and rowdiness of a locker room, and both sides can get teased.

Some girls will tease each other's looks when they change in public. Occasionally, they may also tease the one who chooses more privacy. Try to relax without worrying about what the other girls think, say, or do. We know this can be easier said than done, but remember that girls often tease to deal with their own discomfort. And anytime you're getting naked, privacy is not a bad idea.

Speaking of locker rooms, when you change clothes with other girls, you may notice the tendency to compare yourself with how other girls look. You may wonder, *Are my breasts too big, or are they too small?* And because of our culture's influence, here's what often happens: If they're small, you want them bigger, and if they're large, you wish they were smaller. Sound familiar?

Breasts: An Architectural Feat

Did you know that the human breast is a work of art? It's true. Just like a rose begins with a small bud, the human breast starts with a tiny bud and grows into a mature breast that's fully equipped to nurture a growing baby. The breast continues to change throughout a woman's reproductive years, forming a complex system of lobes and ducts that house and transport milk through the nipple. Isn't that neat?

During your menstrual cycle, your breasts are changing too. Just like the uterus is getting ready for a possible pregnancy, the breasts get ready too.

During the first part of your menstrual cycle, the milk ducts in your breasts grow as estrogen is released. In the second part of your cycle, after ovulation, progesterone rises and milk glands form. As these glands enlarge in the second half of your monthly cycle, your breasts may feel "lumpy." This is normal.

These hormonal effects likely explain the soreness or swollen feeling of your breasts, especially right as your period begins each month.

As your period starts, your breasts return to their normal size, and the whole cycle begins again next month.

Are you starting to recognize that your body is magnificent, beautifully and wonderfully made for God's purposes? Your breasts are another reminder of the gift of your body — God's masterpiece.

Breasts don't simply add curves to a girl's body. If you become a mom one day, you'll have the wonderful opportunity to breastfeed your baby. Breastfeeding provides the best and healthiest milk a baby can have, and that's pretty amazing.

What do you think about all this? God gave you *your* body for a reason, and you're still growing and changing. Embrace yourself just how God made you; appreciate his design for you. Thank him for who you are, whose you are, and who you will become.

Even the Scriptures use a bit of humor and poetry to describe your changing body. Take a look:

> Your breasts are like two fawns, like twin fawns of a gazelle.
>
> *Song of Solomon 7:3*

> Your stature is like that of the palm, and your breasts like clusters of fruit.
>
> *Song of Solomon 7:7*

One last thing: when it comes to your breasts, dressing modestly will help keep the stares off, which will make this transition go more smoothly for you. Pretty soon, you'll get used to your new twin gazelles, and they'll remind you of the precious gift of your femininity.

QUESTION 16

When do I get to shave my legs and underarms?

M y (Dr. Mari's) daughter is a girly girl. Although lately she's grown to love the whole spectrum of the rainbow, for years she's been all about pink and purple, and now she favors blue. Her bedroom is a definite girl zone, featuring the likes of Rapunzel and a host of Pixie Hollow fairies. It's another world in there—magical and mystical.

We love doing things together—from crafts to chats to cuddles. Recently my daughter and I started our own foot soaking tradition. If she needs some cheering up, I invite her to soak her feet with me. She lights up right away. Somehow, as the soapy, warm water hits her feet, her lips get going. We laugh, joke around, and chitchat about everything. I love the opportunity to hear her questions and help her as much as I can—with big and small things.

As you walk through puberty, you too have many questions. You may wonder things like when you can start shaving or when it is appropriate to start wearing makeup. Talk to your mom or another trusted adult about all this. Your friends have their own families, and their viewpoint and rules might be different from yours.

In general, most girls begin shaving between the ages of nine and sixteen. There is quite a bit of variation here, and you can choose not to shave too. This is not a medical necessity by any means; it is more of a cultural and family decision. In some cultures, women shave their underarms and lower legs, but not their thighs. In others, women don't shave at all.

One thing to keep in mind is that, once you start shaving, your hair will grow back differently in that area. It will be less smooth and more prickly. The most important thing is not so much when to shave, but to get permission from your parents before picking up that razor.

Your mom might mention different choices you have, like a handheld razor, an electric razor, or hair-removing cream. She will teach you never to shave your legs while they're dry; that can cause a lot of itching, discomfort, and even a rash. Also, if you're going to swim in the ocean, shave the day before, or your legs will likely start burning as soon as they touch the water. Ouch!

Waxing is not as convenient as shaving, but you can be hair-free for weeks, or longer. Your mom or trusted adult can help you pick out the right wax at any convenience store and help you use it correctly. Read the directions carefully, test it on a small part of your body (to make sure you're not allergic to it), and wait at least six hours before you proceed.

Around the time when your breasts begin to grow, you'll likely notice some hair in the pubic area as well. This usually happens after your breasts bud, but a few girls get pubic hair before their

Will My Hair Grow Thicker After I Shave?

In a word, no! As it grows, each hair tapers, getting thinner at the ends. This is why longer hair bends more easily than shorter hair. This can sometimes lead to those *split ends* you're so glad to get rid of after a haircut.

This is also why shorter hair feels more stubbly than longer hair. The blunt end of shaved hair may feel temporarily coarser, but it's not because it was shaved, but because it's shorter. It's all part of how God made hair.

breasts grow. At first, this hair will be smooth and fine, but as it fills in, it will become coarser and curlier. A year or two after your pubic hair appears, expect to see some hair show up under your arms as well. Woo-hoo.

Through all these changes, make sure you get your mom's or a trusted adult's permission *and* help before shaving anything, especially near your groin (along the inner thighs). Girls don't really need to shave there at all, but some choose to so hair won't show when wearing a bathing suit. Be super careful!

Shaving this sensitive area with a razor can lead to tough-to-treat skin infections that can grow into painful bumps called *boils*—we don't recommend it. And if you do it incorrectly, it can be quite uncomfortable. Using a safe, hair-removing product might be a better alternative at your age, though it's probably best to leave that hair alone.

Remember that, although it's great to talk to your girlfriends, they're learning too, so their answers aren't always correct. If in doubt, ask your mom, an older sister, or a trusted woman. They went through everything you're going through—and more.

QUESTION 17

Get me off this roller coaster. Why am I so moody?

See if this sounds familiar. You wake up full of energy. You put on your favorite shirt, cute shorts, and matching socks, and head to the kitchen for breakfast. As you sit down to eat, your little sister spills her milk and your mom asks you to clean it up.

Without warning and for no good reason, you blow up. Your sister starts crying. Your mom sighs. And your brother walks in, still half asleep, to quite a scene. He burps loudly, and you greet him by yelling at him for sleeping when he could have been helping.

Not a great way to start a morning, is it? But this is exactly the kind of chaos that moodiness can create. Nobody likes it, including you.

Moodiness can mean that one moment you're skipping along, feeling happy, and the next instant you're a grump. Ever feel such contrasting emotions in the same day, even within the same five-minute period? Welcome to puberty.

As a young woman on your journey through puberty, your mood can change in a matter of seconds. You can go from gentle swan to ferocious tigress without so much as a blink. These ever-changing moods can be explained, in part, by a word you're starting to love — *hormones*.

Yes, the same hormones that God designed to guide puberty can also make you moody. But here's the thing. You can't blame everything you feel on these chemicals, and you can't let moods run your life.

Although hormones can make you feel like you're riding an out-of-control emotional roller coaster, we have good news for you. Regardless of how you *feel*, you can control how you respond. God equipped your body with hormones and your spiritual life with fruit:

> The fruit of the Spirit is love, joy, peace, patience, kindness, goodness, faithfulness, gentleness, self-control; against such things there is no law.
>
> *Galatians 5:22–23, NASB*

When life feels out of control, you can choose to exercise *self-control*. And God-given self-control is more powerful than *any* hormone.

I (Dr. Mari) wonder if God gave women hormone shifts partly to help us learn to *exercise* our self-control. You see, regardless of your circumstances or feelings, you *always* have a choice. You can hop off the roller coaster, or at least slow it down, and gain some control over your life.

Here's what can happen when you stay on that loopy roller coaster — it happened to me (Dr. Mari) when I was about twelve.

Before Christmas, my brother and I checked the mail every day, eager to get our favorite toy catalog. One year, it finally came, and he got to it first. Bummer. I waited and waited, and he wouldn't give it up.

I asked nicely again and again, but he refused to share. So what did I do? I stomped out of the room and slammed my bedroom door — WHAM! Everyone heard me, probably even the neighbors. And then someone came to my door.

Still fuming, and certain it was my brother, I let him have it, yelling out words that I can't repeat here. It wasn't pretty. When I finally stopped yelling, I saw my father standing there shocked — and not at all amused. He had kindly brought the catalog and planned to serve it with a smile. Big oops!

When you feed your moods and emotions rather than try to manage them, you end up feeling worse. Sometimes you hurt others too. Has that ever happened to you?

The good news is that, although some moodiness is a normal part of going through puberty, you don't have to live by how you *feel*. You can live by what you *know*. And you know that kindness is better than rudeness and respect is better than rebellion.

So when you wake up feeling down, when you're upset or angry, you have a choice to make. You can exercise self-control in any situation. You can stop yourself before saying something hurtful. You can think *before* you say or do something you might regret. You can regroup, gather your thoughts, and decide if that's the wise and godly choice or not.

It also helps to remember that most bad moods don't last long, so be patient with yourself. Count to ten; maybe take some deep breaths. Walk away — quietly, without stomping — and talk to God about how you feel.

If you need to, have a good, cleansing cry. Go hang out with a cheerful friend, or laugh with your goofy little brother. Read a good book, turn up some good music, and pray. Perhaps you can call a friend or talk to your mom or sister or a funny neighbor.

You can go for a run or a walk or pet your dog. Doing something nice for someone else may help take your mind off yourself. Next thing you know, you're feeling better.

It's important to recognize that, whereas some moodiness is normal, being irritable all the time or very often can signal a problem. If moods get to be too much, and if you also feel extremely tired, sad, or hopeless, you may be getting depressed. If you feel down often or stop enjoying life, talk to your mom or dad or a trusted teacher or adult who can help you. You may need to see a counselor, psychologist, or doctor if these feelings don't go away. We talk much more about depression in the next question.

All the healthy habits we've discussed can help keep your stress level down and balance your moods. And speaking of stress, puberty can be a time of significant stress from school, family, and relationships—and even from your body changes. You may feel like more is expected of you now, and you're right. But you can make this transition smoother and minimize stress.

Did you know that a certain level of stress is good? It energizes you and helps prepare you for what you need to do. But stress that isn't managed well can drain your energy and make you procrastinate and worry. As you learn to use stress to your advantage, you will benefit from the stress hormones that motivate you while minimizing the stress effects that drain you.

So what can you do to cope with stress? As with managing moodiness, eating a healthy diet, staying active, and getting enough rest are critical. Thankfully, there are many fun ways to manage stress. Usually they involve doing the stuff you love to do.

Do you like to sing or dance? Do you love to run? Do you feel better when you're outside surrounded by nature? Make sure you do some of these things you love every day; you will feel happier and less stressed.

When I (Dr. Mari) was twelve, my best friend gave me a journal I've kept all these years. If I felt confused or sad, I would write about it. I felt better and I learned more about myself. Writing

Stressed, Moody, Tired — or All of the Above?

The word *hormone* comes from the Greek word *hormo*, meaning "to set in motion." Hormones set many things into motion, including your metabolism, your growth and development, and, yes, your mood. Hormones like estrogen, serotonin, and beta-endorphins can contribute to a "good mood." Sometimes it's all about hormones, but not always.

Many young people visit their doctor because they feel tired. They lack energy and wonder if something's wrong with their bodies. For most of the girls with these types of complaints, the solution is clear. They need to make better choices. Most of them need:

- *More sleep.* Most tweens and teens need at least nine to ten hours every night (read more about how to get a better night's sleep in question 6).

- *More physical activity.* Exercise gives you energy and speeds up your metabolism (that means your body's wide awake). It also helps you burn fat for energy instead of muscle. And staying physically active helps you feel better during the day and sleep better at night.

- *Better nutrition* (you can read more about this in questions 7 and 10).

- *More fiber.* A high-fiber diet helps you have more energy throughout the day. High-fiber foods include nuts, whole grains, fruits, vegetables, oatmeal, corn, beans, avocados, and others.

- *Less soda and caffeine.* Sugary drinks and caffeine (found in many "energy drinks") can dehydrate you. They remove too much fluid from your body, making you tired. They provide no nutrition at all, only empty calories. Choose water instead.

- *Less bad fats.* A diet high in bad, or *saturated*, fats can slow down your metabolism (your body takes a nap) and make you sluggish. Bad fats can also increase your risk for obesity, heart problems, and diabetes. Instead, consider good fats such as *monounsaturated* fats (found in olive oil, canola oil, sunflower oil, avocados, and nuts) or *polyunsaturated* fats (found in soybean oil, walnuts, sunflower/sesame/pumpkin seeds, flaxseed, fatty fish [salmon, tuna, mackerel, herring, trout, sardines], and soy milk).

- *Stress management.* If stress is not handled properly, it can affect how you feel, how well you do in school, and your relationships. It can make you tired, anxious, or depressed. If you feel stressed out, get help from your parents, teachers, school counselor, and/or a psychologist.

- *No smoking, alcohol, or drugs* (you can read more about these in question 29). All these substances contribute to moodiness, depression, fatigue, anxiety, poor sleep, and countless other problems. Be wise and stay away from all that.

Controlling Your Moodiness

Here are some tips for moody teens from WebMD:

- Think about something or someone you are thankful for.
- Do something nice. It's hard to be in a bad mood when you're helping someone.
- Listen to some upbeat and uplifting music.
- Realize that you're not alone. Talk to a friend about your moods. It might surprise you to discover that others are going through the same mood swings as you.
- Don't keep your feelings to yourself. This can make problems seem much worse than they actually are. If a friend or parent is not available, talk to a teacher or counselor.
- Do something active. Get outside if you can. Go for a walk, ride your bike, play tennis or another favorite sport. Or just take a deep breath and enjoy the fresh air.
- Get enough sleep every night. Being tired can make you feel gloomy and irritable, and it makes it harder to cope with your moods.

can help you deal with stress and moods. It's also a great way to communicate with your parents about tough or embarrassing topics. Give it a try.

Do you enjoy reading? A good book at the right time can bring peace and comfort, or it can simply be fun. Reading the Bible every day will help you know God and his plans for your life. It will also keep you growing all the fruit of the Spirit.

Your friends can also help you deal with the stresses of life. While in middle school, I (Dr. Mari) grew close to three girl-friends, and we're still like sisters. We've cried together, laughed together, and figured out life's messes together.

Some of the friendships you're making now may last a lifetime. So nurture good friendships starting now. Choose your friends well and treat them with love, kindness, and respect. They will often be the ones who give you the most grace on those moody days that we all face.

> The words of the reckless pierce like swords, but the tongue of the wise brings healing.
>
> *Proverbs 12:18*

> Be completely humble and gentle; be patient, bearing with one another in love.
>
> *Ephesians 4:2*

Emotions and the Bible

Did you ever read the story of Job? It's about a good man who lost everything overnight, including his home, riches, and family. Job was depressed for a long time as he tried to make sense of his new life, his suffering, and God. Three friends tried to help him and failed. But God never failed him.

In his grief, Job said:

> "If only my anguish could be weighed and all my misery be placed on the scales! It would surely outweigh the sand of the seas — no wonder my words have been impetuous."
>
> Job 6:2–3

Impetuous means reckless, hotheaded, saying words one might regret. Job's sadness was so deep that even his friends didn't know how to help him. So Job talked to God, sharing his true feelings rather than denying the awful way he felt.

When God answered, Job gained a whole new perspective. Job felt God's love for him once more and said:

> "My ears had heard of you but now my eyes have seen you."
>
> Job 42:5

Job then forgave his friends, and God blessed him.

When we are moody, we can talk to God (by prayer) and listen to God (by reading his Word). I (Dr. Walt) have found that when I'm moody, the books of Psalms and Proverbs are particularly helpful. Here's what I do:

- I look at the date. For example, when I was writing this, it was the third day of the month.
- Then I read one chapter in the book of Proverbs (there are thirty-one chapters in Proverbs) that matches the date: Proverbs 3.
- Then I read several psalms. I take the day of the month and add thirty, again and again, up to 150 (the total number of psalms). So I would read Psalms 3, 33, 63, 93, and 123.
- With the exception of Psalm 119, the psalms and proverbs are short. So I can read one chapter of Proverbs and five chapters of Psalms in just a few minutes.

Our emotions are not a surprise to God; he made us this way. So trust God with the uncertainties of your life, including the changes that come with puberty. He will never fail you.

QUESTION 18

Can my moods be dangerous?

I (Dr. Walt) saw a young woman in my office about six months ago. I'll call her Sophia. She told me she had not been feeling like herself. She kept feeling worse and worse, and her family and friends began to notice.

Sophia felt unmotivated, like her get-up-and-go had got up and gone. She had trouble with her sleep, both trouble going to sleep (we call that *insomnia*) and trouble staying asleep; she would wake up at all hours during the night. So she felt sleepy all day. Even worse, she didn't enjoy her good friends anymore, or the activities she used to love, like biking and shopping.

This wasn't all. Sophia had always been a good student. But over the last three months her grades dropped like a rock. She couldn't concentrate or think as clearly as before. For the first time in her life, she even forgot to turn in an assignment. She denied using any drugs, and a physical exam and lab work at her student health center were all normal.

She was overeating and gaining weight. But worst of all, she just felt like sitting around all day and crying. "I feel sad all the time, Dr. Walt."

Sophia and her mom hadn't thought of it, but I was pretty sure she had depression.

I asked questions and did some additional tests to rule out other possible causes (like a difficult relationship or a hormone problem), but all the tests came back normal. A depression questionnaire confirmed that she was very depressed.

"I can't be depressed," Sophia insisted. "I thought only old people got depressed. Or people who have a friend die." Sophia was wrong on both counts.

Many people don't understand depression. You see, depression can be both a *symptom* that comes and goes and a *disease* that lingers. Although we all feel depressed (sad, down, or just kinda blah) at times, that does not mean we have the *disease* called *depression*. Moods come and go; full-blown depression stays.

Since depression is so common, let's talk about it. The more you know about it, the more likely that you will be able to help others—and maybe even save someone's life. Here's why.

Depression is a deep sadness and despair (think of Job) as well as discouragement that can last weeks, months, years, or a lifetime. People who are depressed often feel hopeless and inadequate. They can feel such gloom and desperation, they even think about hurting themselves or actually do try to hurt themselves or others. So, yes, depression can be very dangerous.

At any one time, about one in five teens (20 percent) has depressive *symptoms*, like persistent sadness, sleeping problems, and irritability. But when it comes to the *disease*, about 6 to 8 percent of teens have some form of depression at any time.

Signs of Depression

People who are depressed show it in different ways. A person may have three or four of these symptoms or just about the whole list. And, with depression, you can't seem to shake them off — they continue to weigh you down day after day. Here are some of the most common symptoms of depression:

- Sadness that won't go away
- Hopelessness
- Persistent boredom
- Unexplained irritability or crying
- Loss of interest in usual activities
- Eating and/or sleeping more or less than normal
- Difficulty falling asleep, or waking up too early
- Missed school or poor school performance
- Threats or attempts to run away from home
- Outbursts of anger, shouting, complaining
- Reckless behavior
- Self-injury, such as cutting or beating oneself
- Aches and pains that don't get better with treatment
- Social isolation, poor communication
- Extreme sensitivity to rejection or failure
- Thoughts about death or suicide
- Alcohol or drug use

In other words, if you're in the average school, and there are 1,000 kids in your school, over 200 will have depressive *symptoms*, like those listed above, while about sixty to eighty will actually be suffering from the *disease* of depression. Yipes! Think about that the next time your school is gathered in a gym or auditorium.

Before the teen years, equal numbers of boys and girls are depressed. But by age thirteen, a dramatic shift occurs. More than twice as many girls as boys are depressed as teens—and this proportion persists into adulthood. Does anyone know why? Well, it turns out that medical detectives have some clues.

A girl's fluctuating hormones lead to real mood shifts during puberty. Sadness, discouragement, and feeling down are natural human emotions that affect all of us at times, but even more so for girls during puberty. Boys also have these emotions, as expressed in many of King David's psalms, which seem to have been written in times of torment, discouragement, sadness, or downright depression.

> Why, my soul, are you downcast? Why so disturbed within me? Put your hope in God, for I will yet praise him, my Savior and my God.
>
> *Psalm 42:5*

You likely have felt sad after a disagreement, argument, or fight with a family member or friend. You naturally would be down after someone close to you moves away. No doubt you've been discouraged if you've done poorly on an assignment, test, or competition. And something like the death of someone we are extremely close to can lead to the saddest of sadness—grief.

However, and this is key, most of the time we deal with these emotions and, over time, we get over them. They pass. Things get better. This is *not* true about the illness of depression when it's not treated.

As Sophia learned, depression affected more than her emotional health. It affected her energy, motivation, concentration, appetite, sleep, and weight. Worst of all, it kept her from enjoying the good things in life she normally enjoyed so much—such as her hobbies, good meals, and her relationships with God, her family, and her best friends.

Why Do People Get Depressed?

There is rarely a single cause for depression in any one person. Many factors can play a role, including:

- Genetics. You can inherit the tendency to develop depression from family members who had it (even as far back as your great-grandparents).
- Past or ongoing emotional abuse, bullying, or trauma.
- Living in a difficult family or social environment.
- Lack of exercise or light (such as during winter) and not getting enough sleep can make depression more likely.
- Inadequate nutrition from an un- healthy diet and/or eating disorders like bulimia and anorexia (you can read more about eating disorders us- ing this QR code or the URL in our resources list).

  National Eating Disorders Association

- Alcohol and/or drug use.
- Many medical disorders can cause or coexist with depression.
- People who are pessimistic (negative — think Eeyore) or melancholic (naturally sad or pensive) can be more prone to depression.
- Sometimes a person can become depressed for no obvious reason at all.

Regardless of the contributing factors, an imbalance of chemicals in the brain results in depression — chemicals like *serotonin*, *norepinephrine*, and *dopamine*. If these *neurotransmitters* get all out of whack, you may start sounding and acting like Eeyore. Like Charlie Brown on bad days, you may begin to sound like you've lost hope.

She was the perfect example of what we talked about in question 1: If one health wheel is out of alignment, it can affect the other three. Sophia's flat emotional health wheel impacted her physical, relational, and spiritual health wheels.

Sophia was like many of our depressed patients in that she did not even realize she was depressed. Like others we see with depression, she mistakenly began to think of herself as a failure, a bad person, a poor student, a quitter, and a loser. And Sophia's mother thought her daughter just had "a bad attitude" or, even worse, was abusing drugs and not admitting it.

I reassured them that it's very common for depression to go unrecognized. "But now that we know what's wrong," I told them, "we can do something about it." We then talked about all the different ways we could begin to help Sophia get better.

When a girl with depression gets the right care, she can get better. But if depression is not diagnosed and treated, it can get worse—sometimes a lot worse. Left untreated, teen depression dramatically increases the risk of attempting suicide or having thoughts about harming oneself. This is especially true for girls, who are more than twice as likely to attempt suicide as boys. Tragically, suicide is the third leading cause of death in people ages ten to twenty-four.

If you have a friend you think is depressed, encouraging them to get the help they need may literally save their life. The good news is that depression is one of the most treatable diseases. The National Association of School Psychologists says, "Virtually everyone who receives proper, timely intervention can be helped." That means getting the right help at the right time.

This is why we tell people who think they are depressed not to wait to get help while hoping it will go away on its own. And if you or a friend might be depressed, getting help should include both of these:

1. *Get a medical checkup.* Your doctor can check for any health problems that might be causing symptoms of

Help for Depression

Beyond the medicines that are sometimes needed to treat depression, so many things can help the disorder. Here are some of them:

- Counseling and/or therapy, preferably from a Christian mental health expert (counselor, psychologist, or therapist). This can be extremely helpful.

- Daily physical activity such as a brisk walk, a bike ride, jogging, or dancing, especially if done with a friend or exercise buddy.

- Getting outside in daylight and enjoying nature and fresh air can lift your mood.

- Good nutrition. One person with depression might overeat while another has no appetite. It's important to eat plenty of fruits and vegetables, drink plenty of water, and not skip meals.

- Healthy food choices, avoiding bad sugars and bad fats, which can make you sluggish.

- Setting aside time to relax and/or learning stress-reduction skills.

- Playing, petting a dog, or doing fun things with good friends.

- Finding something to laugh about—a funny movie or book perhaps.

- Exercising one's imagination (reading, journaling, painting, drawing, doodling, sewing, writing, dancing, composing music, etc.) to get creative juices flowing and loosen up some positive emotions.

- Sleeping well. Good sleep helps people recover from depression more quickly (you can read more about this in question 6).

- Looking on the bright side. Depression affects normal thinking, making everything seem gloomy, negative, and hopeless. I (Dr. Walt) encourage my patients to make an effort to notice the good things in life. I also encourage them to consider their strengths, gifts, and blessings.

- I (Dr. Walt) tell patients to journal each night about five blessings from that day. Then I have them think about these blessings and pray, thanking God for all of them.

- Setting aside quiet time with God each day — talking to him (through prayer) and listening to him (by reading the Bible).

- Studying what God's Word says about sadness, depression, and grief.

- Memorizing Scripture verses that are meaningful and encouraging.

- Joining (or starting) a small group of trusted Christian friends for fellowship, accountability, and prayer.

- Most of all, it's important to be patient. Depression takes time to heal.

depression. For example, having diabetes or a lazy thyroid gland (*hypothyroidism*) can cause a depressed mood, low energy, and tiredness. *Mononucleosis* (mono) is a viral infection that can also make a person feel very tired and even depressed.

These medical problems mimic depression. They make a person look and feel depressed, but when you treat the medical problem, they feel better. Seeing your doctor and getting help for these conditions can make a huge difference.

2. *Talk to a professional counselor.* When someone has depression, "talk therapy" with a therapist or counselor is usually very helpful (even if your doctor also recommends a medication). Here are just a few of the ways talk therapy helps:

   - A counselor will help people with depression understand the disorder and how it affects their emotions. The counselor may teach them how to journal or put their feelings into words. This can help people feel understood and supported.
   - A Christian counselor will point people to helpful Bible verses and help them understand how God can use depression in their lives (like God used the physical challenges in Kate's life from question 1).
   - A therapist will help people develop a plan to work out problems and overcome the negative or self-critical thinking that feeds depression.
   - A Christian counselor can help people develop more positive and biblical ways of looking at things. This helps them learn to accept themselves, which improves their self-esteem.
   - Therapists help people build the confidence they need to deal with depression.

A Simple Screening Test

A simple, two-question *screening* test helps doctors and counselors identify people who might be depressed. They ask: Over the past two weeks, have you been bothered by either of the following problems?

1. Little interest or pleasure in doing things
2. Feeling down, depressed, or hopeless

If you answer, "Not at all," you likely don't have the disease of depression. If you can't answer, "Not at all" to *both* questions, the next step is to talk to a trusted adult about your feelings. They can help you contact a counselor who can help.

The same week that I (Dr. Walt) wrote the first draft of this question, I saw Sophia and her mother back in my office. They'd done much of what I recommended. In her follow-up visits over six months, she continued to get better.

Thankfully, she went back to feeling and acting like a bubbly teenager. At the end of the visit, I asked, "Sophia, what was the most important thing God taught you during your depression?"

She thought a moment, then smiled. "I learned how to trust and obey him even in my darkest moments. And," she said, smiling gratefully at her mom, "he taught me the importance of my family."

She looked back at me. "And now he's given me a ministry with other girls who are sad and depressed. I've found the Bible is true when it says, 'God is our merciful Father and the source of all comfort. He comforts us in all our troubles so that we can comfort others. When they are troubled, we will be able to give them the same comfort God has given us.'"

"Second Corinthians?" I asked.

She smiled and nodded. "Chapter 1, verses 3 and 4. It's from the New Living Translation. It really speaks to me."

"Me too," I replied. Before they left, we prayed and thanked God for being so faithful and so good.

> Even though I walk through the darkest valley, I will fear no evil, for you are with me; your rod and your staff, they comfort me.
>
> *Psalm 23:4*

> "But I will restore you to health and heal your wounds," declares the LORD.
>
> *Jeremiah 30:17*

QUESTION 19

Acne and tanning — how do I win with my skin?

An old expression says, "Beauty is only skin deep." By now, you know that this is not true from God's perspective. He considers you his beautiful creation because he created you in his image.

Still, most girls have two areas of concern when it comes to their skin: (1) the annoying reality of acne and (2) the *perceived* benefits of tanning. So what do you need to know to have the healthiest skin possible?

Let's start with acne, which is a normal and natural (and, yes, annoying) part of growing up. The primary cause of acne is overactive oil glands in your skin, especially on your face, neck, chest, and back. The same hormones that lead to puberty rev up these oil glands.

Since different girls have different reactions to their hormones, some will get more acne than others. Stress can also worsen acne. But the good news is that there's a lot you can do to reduce the number and severity of breakouts.

You'll be delighted to learn that foods like pizza and chocolate do *not* cause acne. However, it is possible that these foods, dairy products, or diets high in sugars may cause or worsen acne in *some* kids. The American Academy of Dermatology (AAD) says:

- If you think a food might be worsening your acne, consider avoiding that product for a time.
- Be patient. After you start avoiding that food item, it may take up to twelve weeks for your acne to improve.
- If you're convinced that dairy products worsen your acne and decide to limit or avoid them, talk to your doctor or pharmacist about taking a calcium and vitamin D supplement.

An over-the-counter acne medication can often clear up mild breakouts of acne. Look for a product with benzoyl peroxide (BP), a peeling agent that helps clear pores. Here are some of our BP tips:

- Sometimes BP can bleach clothing, so it's better to use it at night.
- Start with a product with 5 percent BP. Apply it at night after washing your face.
- Since BP causes dryness and flaking, use a moisturizing lotion after the BP.
- We recommend lotions instead of creams, as they are less likely to clog your pores. Make sure the lotion is fragrance-free, oil-free, and non-comedogenic.
- After about five days of daily use, if your acne hasn't improved much and your skin isn't irritated, use the 5 percent lotion twice a day. Or you may switch to a lotion with 10 percent BP and use it once a day (at bedtime).

Acne: Save Face

Here are some effective ways to help prevent acne — or at least reduce the number of attacks:

- Keep your skin clean. This helps remove excess oils and dead skin cells that can clog your pores. But washing too much can dry out your skin or irritate existing acne.
- Keep it simple. Wash your face with a moisturizing soap twice a day. Some physicians recommend an antibacterial soap. Ideally, it should be a *noncomedogenic* soap, which means it won't cause or worsen acne.
- Wash your face and body with your hands rather than a washcloth, and never scrub.
- Avoid harsh alcohol-based or oil-based cleansers.
- Wash after exercising; sweat and dirt can clog your pores and worsen acne.
- Gently pat dry with a clean towel.
- Keep hair gel and other hair products away from your face as much as possible. Many hair products contain chemicals that can worsen acne.
- Try not to pick at your face or lean your chin on your hands, which can worsen your breakout.

- After another four to five days of consistent use, if your acne still hasn't improved and your skin isn't irritated, use the 10 percent BP twice a day.

If these tips don't work and your acne does not get better (or if it worsens), see your family's doctor. Your doctor is trained to help get your skin to look its best and probably also dealt with acne as a teen.

Acne will usually improve with simple prescription gels or creams, oral medications, or a combination of both. But you'll need to be very patient. It may take weeks or a few months to find the exact combination of medicines to help clear up your acne. There are many, many options, and one will help, eventually. So don't give up too soon.

While you wait, you may be tempted to squeeze and pop a big pimple. This may actually worsen your acne by pushing the infected material deeper into the skin and causing even more swelling and redness. Popping pimples may even leave a purplish mark that stays on the skin for weeks. Squeezing pimples can also lead to scarring. Don't do it!

The best news of all is that, in general, acne gets better and is often greatly improved or gone by the time you complete puberty. Prescription treatments usually work if you follow your doctor's advice.

Acne isn't the only thing affecting your skin that can show up during puberty. You need to make some very important decisions about tanning—whether in the sun or in a tanning salon.

As I (Dr. Walt) was writing this chapter, I saw a sad news report about a young woman who was told her chance of survival was only 20 percent. As you can imagine, she was devastated. What disease threatened her life? It was a type of skin cancer. But what caused her cancer was the real surprise—the twelve indoor tanning sessions she had just before her wedding day.

Only six years after getting married, this young woman was diagnosed with one of the most dangerous and potentially fatal forms of skin cancer—*melanoma*—and it had spread throughout her body.

More and more women with skin cancer are teaming up to warn young girls like you about the dangers of tanning.

Many of our young patients (and their parents) are shocked to learn that sunburns and tanning are major risk factors for getting skin cancer. In fact, having one or more blistering sunburns as a child or teenager increases your risk of developing skin cancer as an adult. Would you believe that one in two young people reports having had at least one sunburn in the past year?

But not all skin cancers come from outdoor tanning. Many come from indoor tanning.

Most girls believe that sun exposure is good for their health and that tanning salons are perfectly safe. Unfortunately, although many, if not most, tanning salons claim to be healthy and safe, they're not.

Did you know that teens who use indoor tanning beds have a 75 percent increased chance of getting melanoma? And if you tan indoors, your chance of another type of skin cancer — *basal cell carcinoma* — is 69 percent higher than those who never do. No wonder many states and countries have banned the use of indoor tanning devices for those under eighteen.

No wonder the AAP points out that "indoor tanning is a potent source of ultraviolet radiation, especially UVA," which "can be as much as 10 to 15 times more powerful than midday sunlight."

And there's more. Using a tanning bed may become addictive. According to one small study of people who do this often, their brain can look (during a tanning session) like the brain of people on drugs.

Also, indoor or outdoor tanning can cause wrinkles and premature aging. It's true. Tanning can cause both skin cancer *and* wrinkles. Yikes! You can see why we tell people that "no tan is a safe tan."

The bottom line? *No* indoor tanning is safe — especially for kids and teens, whose skin is far more susceptible to these harmful, cancer-causing sources of UV rays.

So what can you do to have healthier skin that's less likely to wrinkle or get skin cancer? Avoid too much sun and all tanning and sunburns. Wear sunscreen when outdoors. This will decrease your risk a lot.

On any given day, if you'll be in the sun for more than fifteen minutes between 9:00 a.m. and 4:00 p.m., wear sunscreen or a moisturizing lotion with ultraviolet (UV sunlight) protection. Remember that it takes at least twenty minutes for the sunscreen to be absorbed into the skin and begin to work.

Look for products with a sun protection factor (SPF) of at least 15 that protects against both damaging types of sun rays — ultraviolet A (UVA) *and* ultraviolet B (UVB) rays. You'll notice that many sunscreen products have an SPF of 45, 50, or even 60. But an SPF greater than 30 offers very little advantage. The difference in skin protection above SPF 15 is minimal. And the higher the SPF, the greater the cost and the greater the risk of adverse effects like a rash or an allergic reaction.

We recommend products with an SPF of 15 or 20 for most girls. But for those who are more sensitive to the sun, an SPF of 30 should be plenty.

Also, the SPF ratings only apply to UVB protection. UVA rays are less likely to burn, but they penetrate deeper into the skin and can lead to wrinkles, sagging, discoloration, and redness or rashes. UVA also contributes to your risk for dangerous forms of skin cancer. That's why we tell our patients to buy a *full* or *broad-spectrum* sunscreen that protects against UVA *and* UVB rays.

How much sunscreen should you apply? According to the American Academy of Dermatology, a heaping handful of sunscreen (at least one to two ounces) should be applied to exposed skin every day — including your face, ears, neck, and arms (as well as your legs or feet if exposed).

And speaking of the sun ... have you noticed you sweat a little more these days? We'll talk about this normal change in the next question.

QUESTION 20

Why do I sweat? It makes me feel like a boy.

Like body hair, sweating is not just for boys. Too bad, right?

The good news is that there are many ways to deal with sweat and its partner, body odor (BO). We're sorry to say it, but girls have BO too. You know, smells that are not terribly pleasant or "feminine," or, to put it bluntly, smells that just stink. There—we've said it. Even girls— cute girls, adorable girls—can be stinky at times.

Of course, it's good and normal to sweat when you're working out or playing. It's part of God's divine design to help cool you down when your body heats up. But normal sweat can get quite stinky. My (Dr. Mari's) son loves telling jokes. He recently asked, "Mom, what do you call a fairy that doesn't take a bath?" You'll love the answer: "Stinker-bell."

Anyway, you can keep the Stinker-bell and sweaty days to a minimum. With just a little help, stink can turn pretty pink in no time. And girls can have more fun with this than boys, since we have so many fragrances and fun products to choose from.

Did you ever shop for body lotions with your mom or girlfriends? You can find balms, lotions, sprays, creams, powders, bubble bath, gels, soaps, and oils. By using only products that are safe for young skin, you can have a lot of fun with these.

You could spend hours exploring all the fragrances and products out there that help make being a girl so fun. There's ginger, lavender, pomegranate, vanilla, and every kind of berry. You can enjoy jasmine and honeysuckle.

Yet, along with beautiful scents, God allows us to have stinky smells and BO, doesn't he? Let's talk about why this happens and how you can prevent it and deal with it.

Sweating is one way the body cools itself down—it's part of the miracle of your perfectly integrated body. And did you know that sweat is actually odorless? Sweat is stink-free until it combines with bacteria that normally live on your skin. So you can blame those pesky germs for stinking up sweat.

The first thing you can do is to dry up. Less sweat means there's less fluid for the bacteria to mix with, which means less odor. Washing your underarms with water and a mild soap every day and after sporting events will always help.

Early in the puberty years you can start using an antiperspirant (which helps you sweat less), a deodorant (which removes and covers up smells), or a product that combines the two. But remember to wash before using deodorant, or you'll just be covering up BO without getting rid of it. You can end up with some very interesting smells that way.

If a traditional deodorant doesn't work well for you, a few products are available without a doctor's prescription that are much stronger. Your pharmacist or doctor's office can recommend one. These products work differently and are usually applied at bedtime. After a few nights of use, daytime sweating usually improves a lot or goes away. You can then continue to use this every other night or as needed to keep sweating under control.

Some people sweat so much that it starts to affect their lives. They may choose white shirts more often to hide sweat marks, or they may not raise their hands in class to hide their embarrassing wetness. Don't let this be you.

If you cannot control sweating from your underarms, palms, or soles, see your doctor to figure out why. Some people sweat more than others. Excessive and unpredictable sweating, called *hyperhidrosis*, is usually hereditary, but occasionally it's related to medical conditions. In most cases, your doctor can prescribe a safe but stronger product that will usually work.

What about stinky feet? In some places, people are expected to leave their shoes at the door when they enter someone's home. This could be embarrassing if your feet smell, but this too can be prevented. Here are some tips:

- Don't wear the same shoes all the time. Let them breathe between wears.
- Wash your feet every day, and avoid wearing wet shoes or sneakers. They can get very stinky when wet, so let them dry out, or ask a parent if the shoes can be thrown in the dryer. Ask first, though; you don't want to ruin the dryer or the shoes.
- It also really helps to wear socks every time you wear closed-toe shoes. If you don't, get ready for a big "phew" moment.
- Sprinkle your shoes and feet with foot powder, which absorbs the wetness that contributes to smelly feet. You can even use antifungal powder. This will help prevent athlete's foot, an itchy fungal infection similar to yeast infections. (You learned about yeast infections in question 14.)

"Tanning" Your Smelly Feet

My (Dr. Walt's) friends Joe and Teresa Graedon, who write for the website *The People's Pharmacy*, have a tip on preventing sweaty feet that I've used with teens for years:

> Sweaty feet can lead to foot odor and increase the risk of athlete's foot. One dermatologist we consulted offered the following home remedy: Boil five tea bags in a quart of water for five minutes. When the solution cools, soak your hands or feet for twenty to thirty minutes nightly.

One day on Oprah's TV show, Dr. Mehmet Oz said, "There are a quarter-million sweat glands on your feet. You can generate about a half a liter of sweat from your foot in a day. It really does make a lot of juice." Like the Graedons, he recommended, "Brew up some mild iced tea and put your feet in it for about thirty minutes a day for a week. The tannic acid in the tea will actually tan your foot a little bit, which will dry it out."

The only catch is that using this treatment can stain the feet a bit — leaving a slight yellow tint on the skin.

You may have heard about *athlete's foot*. It's a common infection of the skin on the feet caused by a germ called *fungus*. People who spend a lot of time wearing sports shoes like cleats, dance shoes, or sneakers get these itchy infections more often. Shoes that don't "breathe" well get moist and sticky on the inside, which helps the fungus overgrow. It also makes your feet get softer and more susceptible to this unwelcome guest. When the fungus overgrows, the web area between your toes gets irritated and uncomfortable and can even crack open.

These infections are one reason I (Dr. Mari) loved growing up in the tropics. When you walk around barefoot, you don't need to worry about athlete's foot. Yes, you're right—you may have to worry about stepping on a rusty nail, sharp rocks, or an open stapler—yep, I did that when I was ten, ouch!

The good news is that athlete's foot is usually easy to treat with over-the-counter creams like *terbinafine* or *clotrimazole*. But it's critical to keep your feet dry so the infection doesn't keep coming back. If it does, see your doctor.

We think that God allows some unpleasant things in our bodies to remind us that we all share some of the same difficulties. Perhaps this helps us all be more compassionate. In 2 Corinthians 12:7 the apostle Paul described a "thorn" in his flesh that he prayed about repeatedly. Still, God chose to let him keep it for a purpose. This thorn reminded Paul that in every circumstance God's grace was enough to get him through it.

So whether you're challenged by sweat, acne, or stinky feet, ask God to help you deal with it. As with Paul, there might be a thing or two you'd rather change but can't. Sweating might be one of those things you'd like to get rid of, or perhaps you'd rather never deal with acne. We understand.

The good news is that with most of these annoying body changes, there is a lot you can do, even on those stinky-and-not-so-girly-pink days.

> Perfume and incense bring joy to the heart, and the pleasantness of a friend springs from their heartfelt advice.
>
> *Proverbs 27:9*

QUESTION 21

What's the big deal about modesty?

My (Dr. Mari's) family was leaving Disney World when my seven-year-old daughter, Hannah, began to sing and twirl. I asked what she was singing. She replied softly, "Mami, faith dresses me and makes me beautiful in God's eyes. That's what my song is about."

Yes, I thought. *You're right.*

Hannah's song hints at something wonderful — she knows that God's love is the source of true beauty. As she loves him back, she begins to see herself through his eyes. That is beautiful.

Here's what amazes me about the song of my daughter's heart. She sang about true beauty while surrounded by princesses dressed the part. I mean, who doesn't love to look at Cinderella and Belle? Their dresses are gorgeous, and their feminine grace makes them look even better.

Yet, while admiring them, my daughter thought, "Faith dresses me and makes me beautiful in God's eyes." Her song reminds me of these words from the Bible:

> So in Christ Jesus you are all children of God through faith, for all of you who were baptized into Christ have clothed yourselves with Christ.
>
> *Galatians 3:26–27*

> I delight greatly in the LORD; my soul rejoices in my God. For he has clothed me with garments of salvation and arrayed me in a robe of his righteousness, as a bridegroom adorns his head like a priest, and as a bride adorns herself with her jewels.
>
> *Isaiah 61:10*

Rather than focus on your outward clothes, it's critical to first think about what you're wearing on the inside—what clothes your heart.

God loves you just as you are. But do you feel like you're dressed with Christ's love and acceptance? This inner clothing is essential to why modesty matters. Talking about outer looks apart from this understanding makes modesty seem like one more annoying rule to follow. It is far from that.

The desire and willingness to dress modestly comes from the heart that knows its most important clothing is on the inside—God's love and acceptance.

Our deepest desire is that, while reading this book, you will recognize that you've been called to be a princess who is loved, accepted, and embraced by an awesome King.

Did you know that you already have your own Prince Charming? His name is Jesus. Your Prince loves you so much that he

Naked and Spiritually Dead, Dressed and Inwardly Alive

In the Garden of Eden, Eve chose to listen to the serpent, and Adam chose to listen to Eve. Neither one listened to God. After Adam and Eve sinned, they suddenly realized they were naked. Until then, it had not even fazed them. Yet after choosing their way over God's way, they felt ashamed of their nakedness. So they made some clothes from fig leaves and hid. And do you know what God did?

Even though they had sinned and rebelled against him, God still clothed them. He made even better clothes for them than they had made for themselves. His were leather garments — made to last (at least compared to leaves).

God did not want his creation dressed in guilt and shame. Even though they'd just slapped God in the face, he was merciful and made new clothes just for them.

In the same way, Jesus died on the cross to take our sin upon himself and dress us in his righteousness — his goodness and grace. The Sinless One took up our sin and gave those who follow him a new heart — a clean heart. That awesome gift is available to you as well.

Do you want this inner clothing, this new heart? Then ask Jesus, now, if you'd like, to clothe you in his righteousness. He will. In his goodness and love he will send his Holy Spirit to live in you and to change you from the inside out. And there is no better wardrobe than this.

> "I will give them an undivided heart and put a new spirit in them; I will remove from them their heart of stone and give them a heart of flesh."
>
> Ezekiel 11:19

rushed into this world to battle for you. He came to rescue you. He fought a mighty enemy and gave his life for you. For *you*.

This Prince considers you worthy of his love and his tender care. To him, you are worth more than diamonds and rubies — you are priceless. His life wasn't too high a price to pay. To this Prince, you are beautiful, precious, and one in a billion, since it's estimated that just over one billion humans have lived on the earth since the dawn of time.

God's love, the source of your inner beauty, can become the driving force of your life. It can wake you up every morning and guide every choice you make. Here's what can happen:

You recognize that the one who created you loves you like no one else. He knows your thoughts, including what you like about yourself and what you don't. He knows your every secret. He knows every good and bad thought you have. He knows you intimately. And, knowing you, he loves every bit of you — from the top of your head to the tips of your toes.

The more you recognize how much he loves you, the more you want to live according to his best plans for you. Little by little, the choice to delight God above all else affects everything you do — the music you choose to hear, the movies you watch, what you say and do — even what you think.

One of these choices involves the way you look on the outside — in particular, the clothes you wear, the makeup and jewelry you wear, even the words you use. The way you present yourself to others says something about who you are, what you want, what you care about — and, most important, whose you are. It also impacts how others perceive and treat you. So modesty is not simply about rules that say do this and don't do that.

> Charm is deceptive, and beauty is fleeting; but a woman who fears the LORD is to be praised.
>
> *Proverbs 31:30*

Pure Fashion

Pure Fashion encourages teen girls to live, act, and dress according to their dignity as children of God. They focus on guiding girls ages fourteen to eighteen "to become confident, competent leaders who live the virtues of modesty and purity in their schools and communities." Their goal is "to show the public that it is possible to be stylish, cute, and MODEST."

Pure Fashion writes:

We understand that many young women today are losing their sense of innocence at a very young age, and Pure Fashion aims to reverse this trend by offering a fun, exciting and effective program.

Pure Fashion is a character formation program that enhances not only a young woman's external appearance, but more important, her interior beauty and balanced self-confidence.

You can learn more about Pure Fashion using the URL in our resources list at the back of the book.

She is clothed with strength and dignity; she can laugh at the days to come. She speaks with wisdom, and faithful instruction is on her tongue.

Proverbs 31:25–26

We love the verses from Proverbs 31. They describe a woman of virtue. She is "clothed with strength and dignity," and "she speaks with wisdom." She reminds me (Dr. Mari) of the most influential woman in my life: my mother, Mami. She was beautiful — inside and out — like Esther. She was generous, loving, and kind, and she had a servant heart. She loved to laugh and she loved helping others. Her quiet strength and dignity came through in the way she spoke, walked, and dressed. Everything about her radiated confidence, beauty, and strength.

Mami exemplified modesty and made it fun. She loved jewelry, accessories, and nice clothes. Her wardrobe was full of cute blouses, sparkly pins and belts, and, of course, awesome shoes.

We already pointed out how the feminine grace with which you carry yourself enhances the way you look. This is how Mami was. Her inner beauty and dignity made everything she wore more beautiful. Her clothes didn't have to be expensive, sexy, or glamorous to look great. She knew you don't need to show a bunch of skin to look beautiful.

When it comes to feminine grace, Mami was my Cinderella. No, she did not wear evening gowns to the mall. But everything about her taught me about modesty and true beauty.

So what is this dress called *modesty* that true beauty wears?

Modesty is about showing good judgment and restraint. Modesty makes you avoid what's indecent and favor what's appropriate. Granted, what's acceptable, trendy, and cool is often defined by the culture we live in. But God's principles define what's right and proper for girls.

QUESTION 22

Clothing, thoughts, and good choices — what's the connection?

In the last question, we laid a foundation for why modesty matters. If you haven't read question 21, please read it now before you go on; that background is too important. Here are three important reasons why modesty matters:

1. It affects you.
2. It affects others.
3. It affects your relationship with God.

Why? Let's look at how the Bible views modesty:

> I also want the women to dress modestly, with decency and propriety, adorning themselves, not with elaborate hairstyles or gold or pearls or expensive clothes, but with good deeds, appropriate for women who profess to worship God.
>
> *1 Timothy 2:9–10*

Again, that doesn't mean that all jewelry, accessories, and attractive clothing are out. Not at all. It means that your inner beauty is *most* important. It also emphasizes that, when excessive or inappropriate, clothing and jewelry can be a distraction. They can cause you and others to focus on the wrong things.

God calls us to honor him in our hearts, in our minds, and with our bodies. If your body is for God, and God for your body, then what dress is appropriate for you? That which is proper and decent. Clothing that is dignified and not revealing, that shows you respect yourself and others, and that guards the gift of your sexuality.

Modesty is about recognizing the gift of being a girl and becoming a woman. As you keep reading, ask your mom or a trusted adult questions. The need for modesty exists partly because you are not only a spiritual being, but a relational, sexual person. What does that mean?

Here's a bit of background. The Bible teaches that when we ask Jesus to live and reign in our hearts, when we become followers of Jesus, we become a temple of God's Holy Spirit.

> Do you not know that your bodies are temples of the Holy Spirit, who is in you, whom you have received from God? You are not your own.
>
> *1 Corinthians 6:19*

Why is that word *temple* used? A temple is a place that is sacred, holy, *set apart* for a special purpose. God is telling you that he has set your body apart as the home of his Spirit — to live there — within you. That is a very big deal. So you want to treat your body in a *very* special way.

Your body is an important part of God's divine design for you. As you grow older and if God ordains it, his plan for you may include the opportunity to get married. You may then be blessed to bring a child into the world. Through your body, you can participate in the miracle of a new life. Wow!

Your body, amazing as it sounds, has been reserved for one man — if God calls you to marry. If not, then your body is set apart for God, and God alone. Thinking about your body in this way will impact the way you treat your body, which includes how you dress.

Just as you might like someone's wit, sense of humor, or loving personality, you might also like how someone looks, right? While in high school, I (Dr. Mari) saw a boy who was so gorgeous he took my breath away. As he walked by our lunch table, I had a brilliant idea. "Hey, girls, a moment of silence ... here comes Pete." Our chatter paused as the five of us admired him. Then one sighed, another giggled — and we all burst into laughter.

Finding boys attractive is, of course, completely normal. In fact, it is part of God's design for relationships and marriage that girls find boys handsome and boys find girls cute. Because of this natural attraction between boys and girls, modesty is not just about you. It is also about caring for others, because the way you dress will impact the boys who see you.

Boys and men are very visual. That's just how their brains are wired. Dressing sexy can make a boy focus on your looks so much that it's distracting. It can make him start thinking about wanting to kiss or hug when you're just trying to talk. Dressing immodestly can lead him to focus on your body rather than *all* that you are — inside and out.

Here's an example. Suppose a girl chooses to wear a really tight shirt that shows lots of cleavage. She then starts talking to a boy at school. She shares about her trip to the beach while the young man, trying to be respectful, fights the urge to stare at her chest and down her shirt.

If he cares about guarding his eyes, his mind, and his heart for his future wife, he'll try hard to look into the girl's eyes, but her choice of clothing can make this much more difficult. He'll have to work to listen to her story. Her clothing actually makes it harder for him to see and appreciate who she is.

"Who Says It Has to be Itsy-bitsy?"

I (Dr. Mari) recently watched a video where actress Jessica Rey shares the story of the bikini and why she decided to design her own line of swimwear. Her goal is to "disprove the age-old notion that, when it comes to swimsuits, less is more ... You can dress modestly without sacrificing fashion." Her inspiration was Audrey Hepburn, who is "timeless and classy" and dressed very modestly. "I don't think people think of Audrey Hepburn and think frumpy, dumpy, and out of fashion."

Rey goes on to explain that "modesty isn't about covering up our bodies because they're bad. Modesty isn't about hiding ourselves. It's about revealing our dignity."

Reminding girls and women that we were made beautiful — in God's image and likeness — she ends with this challenge, *"How will you use your beauty?"* Check out the video and her swimsuit designs using this QR code.

Jessica Rey
Swimwear

Imagine a painting with a fancy frame that is so overdone, the frame takes your attention away from the painting. You end up admiring the frame rather than the work of art. It's the same idea. Your outer appearance is like a frame that either distracts from or enhances your inner beauty. Which will it be?

Of course, you are *not* responsible for others' thoughts, but how you dress can contribute to those thoughts. And the Bible gives you this instruction:

> Make up your mind not to put any stumbling block or obstacle in the way of a brother or sister.

Romans 14:13

Again, you are *not* responsible for the way others choose to act in response to how you look. But your outer appearance is like a traffic light. The way you dress can be like a red light that says, "I respect myself and you, and I know there's much more to me than my looks."

Also, the Bible teaches, "In humility value others above yourselves, not looking to your own interests but each of you to the interests of others" (Philippians 2:3 – 4). I (Dr. Walt) can tell you that many guys would greatly appreciate your help by not presenting them with unnecessary temptation.

In one survey, 97 percent of Christian teen boys said they believe that girls and women can dress attractively while being modest. They agreed with the statement that guys definitely notice and appreciate when a woman dresses modestly.

So you can help boys out and respect yourself by wearing appropriate clothing. Of course, you are free, in most schools, to wear what you want. But what's allowed and what's best are totally different choices.

Modesty also means that you dress your age. Experts warn that girls whose clothing, accessories, and makeup make them look older are at greatest risk for sexual sin. And a study by psychologists found that girls who dress older than their age or who dress sexy are more likely to have eating disorders, low self-esteem, and depression.

So modesty matters, but it's not simply one more rule to follow. It's also not about being ashamed of your body. Not at all. The body God gave you is a beautiful gift. Modesty is about loving God and wanting to honor him with your choices. It's about valuing and treating your body — and others — with respect.

I (Dr. Walt) was so happy to hear about the courage of high-school freshman Saige Hatch. In 2012 she organized what is said to be the first modesty club in America at South Pasadena High School in California.

Saige told one reporter that she was sick of seeing her peers

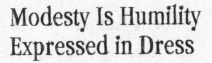

Modesty Is Humility Expressed in Dress

Jenni Smith writes in the GirlTalk blog, "Modesty is humility expressed in dress, a desire to serve others, neither promoting nor provoking sensuality or lust." The Women of Spirit blog says, "The essence of modesty is not setting rules about skirt length, but living a life that brings glory to God rather than ourselves. Dressing to show off is a huge temptation for many women."

Did you ever wonder what boys think about how girls dress? In a study that surveyed 1,600 Christian boys, most of them said that skimpy skirts and bikinis are not modest. Most boys (70 percent) felt that showing any cleavage is immodest. What about pants with words across the rear end? A big no-no. What about low-cut tops layered with more modest shirts? Most of the boys felt these were all right. Formfitting skirts? About evenly split.

You can find more of the results of The Modesty Survey with the URL in our resources list at the back of the book.

revealing too much skin when she came to school each day. She was surprised at her fifteen-year-old friends wearing midriff-grazing tops and short shorts, while exposing their cleavage.

A statement on her club's website says, "A shift is coming, sneaking through the literal fabric of our culture. Our bright heroic women are being made the fool. A fool to think that to be loved they must be naked. To be noticed they must be sexualized," or dress sexy.

Saige writes, "I noticed from elementary school to middle school, and now in high school, a lot of girls were dressing

Secret Keeper Girls

Author Dannah Gresh encourages girls to keep the secrets of their God-given beauty for their future husband. Check out these cool Truth or Bare Fashion Tests from her website, which you can find with the URL in our list of resources:

1. How short is too short? Sit in front of a mirror — crisscross your legs if in shorts, or sit in a chair with your legs crossed if wearing a skirt. If your underwear or a lot of thigh flashes you in the mirror, those shorts or skirt are too short. Give them to your little sister and go shopping for new ones with Mom.

2. What about your shirt? If a lot of chest skin shows up in the mirror when leaning forward, that shirt fails the modesty test. You want to keep all that beauty to share with your future husband, not everyone at school. Consider layering shirts (with a tank top underneath) or wearing a different one.

For more tips, including how to shop for fun, attractive, modest swimwear, visit Dannah's website, secretkeepergirl. com. You can also learn about their cool pajama parties for girls and moms. Secret Keeper Girls surround themselves with wise friends who, like them, believe God's definition of beauty and choose to live a godly life for him. They help each other keep making right choices, they value modesty, and they love to have fun.

Also, ask your mom to get a copy of Dannah's book, *8 Great Dates for Moms and Daughters.* I (Dr. Walt) especially liked taking my daughter on the "tea date." For me (Dr. Mari), tea parties at home are weekly opportunities to have fun, laugh, and talk about beauty, modesty, and lots more with my daughter. Check out Dannah's book using our resources list at the back of this book.

immodestly. I wanted to bring awareness and remembrance to the value of modesty."

Her Modesty Club website, which you can find with this QR code or with the URL in our list of resources, now has members from all fifty states and fourteen countries. They agree with these modesty club standards:

Modesty Club

- If it's too tight, it's not quite right.
- Shoulders and busts are graciously covered.
- Revealing lines are warning signs.
- When I pass this test, I'll be dressed for success.

Have fun with the way you dress, but remember that a pure heart is more beautiful than any clothing you'll *ever* wear.

And don't judge others simply by how they look. It is possible for a girl who wants to be pure but hasn't learned about modesty to dress in a way that looks sexy. It is also possible for a girl to dress modestly and harbor impure thoughts. Most people learn how to dress from their families and culture, and there's quite a bit of peer pressure to look trendy, sexy, and cool.

This might be the first time you've heard this topic presented in this way. So from now on, consider your choices in light of God's call to modesty. Talk to your parents after reading this together if you have questions about what's considered appropriate for you. Before choosing your wardrobe, ask yourself, *What will the way I dress say about me—who I am, whose I am, what I care about, and how I see others and myself?*

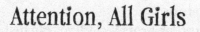

Attention, All Girls

Consider this poignant appeal we've seen on several social media websites:

Dear Girls,

Dressing immodestly is like rolling around in manure. Yes, you'll get attention, but mostly from pigs.

Sincerely,
Real Men

Before you dress, we pray that your heart will sing, "God's love dresses me and makes me beautiful in his eyes!"

Like a gold ring in a pig's snout is a beautiful woman who shows no discretion.

Proverbs 11:22

QUESTION 23

So we all have body hair — some of it we shave off, while some of it we keep, enjoy, and style.

I (Dr. Mari) will never forget my neighbor growing up. She was a cute girl with long, straight hair. One day she returned home after a haircut and perm, and Mami and I heard screams coming from her bedroom. We listened in and heard her cry out, "This is the worst day of my life, Mom. I hate my hair."

This was her first attempt at a perm, and I'm pretty sure she never tried it again.

Her story may sound silly, but you know what I'm talking about. There's just something about girls and hair. And here's what I've noticed: Girls with naturally curly hair (like me)

157

sometimes long for straight hair, and girls with straight hair want curls and waves.

When Mami and I saw my neighbor's hair, we thought it looked really cute. Still, she went back and had it cut even shorter, and complained about her new hairstyle that whole month. Perhaps it helps to remember that we all have bad hair days, and, thankfully, hair always grows back. At least it did for my daughter when, at age three, she cut off a clump of her hair while pretending to be Mulan.

Whether you have naturally wavy or straight hair, enjoy different hairstyles and have fun with your hair. From braids to bows to hairbands, styling your hair can be a wonderful way to enjoy your femininity and spend fun time together with your mom and girlfriends.

Different hairstyles can be so much fun. If you have natural curls, we recommend a book called *Curly Girl: The Handbook*, by Michelle Massey and Lorraine Bender. It's full of great tips to nurture your curls and help you manage frizz. Read it when you wake up with a lion's mane. A good book for all hair types is American Girl's *Hair-Styling Tips and Tricks for Girls*. Check out Tips and Tricks using this QR code or the URLs in our resources list at the back of the book.

Hair-Styling Tips and Tricks for Girls

One thing we see often, especially in girls with lots of hair, is a flaky scalp. This is very common and often related to not scrubbing your scalp well enough when you shampoo. Just like the skin on your body, your scalp cells are constantly being turned over. Since your hair is in the way, your scalp skin needs extra scrubbing to remove those dead skin cells. Lovely thought, isn't it?

If scrubbing doesn't remove all the flakiness, try some over-the-counter dry skin or dandruff shampoo. If the problem persists, talk to your doctor.

So what about makeup? The first thing is this. Although makeup can be fun to wear, remember where your true beauty comes from. Girls look best with a natural look without excessive makeup.

Wearing too much makeup can make you look older, which is not such a good idea. Don't let the culture's obsession with outer beauty steal your innocence and push you to grow up too fast. Enjoy being your age—it will only come once.

Speaking of your face, did you know that young girls and teens have sensitive skin? It's important to treat your face gently, as you learned in question 19. One way to be gentle with your face is by not overdoing it with makeup and products that may irritate your skin. Be careful how you treat your face, and it will smile back at you.

As far as painting your nails, here's what I (Dr. Mari) have noticed: Many moms let their girls paint their toenails earlier than their fingernails. In our home, experimenting with fun, multi-color shades is for little toes. For fingernails, we keep it simple, using lighter shades and less striking colors. This has worked well for us but, again, different families have their own guidelines. Make sure you know what's acceptable in your family. But remember to always present yourself in a way that honors God and reveals your self-respect and dignity.

> You are altogether beautiful, my darling; there is no flaw in you.
>
> *Song of Solomon 4:7*

> "And why do you worry about clothes? See how the flowers of the field grow. They do not labor or spin."
>
> *Matthew 6:28*

Diamonds or sterling —
are body piercings bad?

Body piercing and tattooing are all the rage. It's hard to find a celebrity or sports star without one or both, or a lot of both. We bet you know more than one girl who has expressed her independence and personal style with a piercing.

What you won't find are very many girls who know the risks of body piercing. In fact, when I (Dr. Walt) talk to girls your age, less than one in twenty is aware of the risks. We want you to be smart. You may even help your friends make some wise decisions.

Did you know that body piercing is illegal for minors in almost every state? There are many good reasons for this.

Unlike hair and nail shops, which are strictly regulated by each state, body-piercing shops are pretty much unregulated in

America. With little or no regulation, shop owners don't have to answer to anyone about the safety of their procedures and equipment. They have little incentive to protect you and your friends against infections and other health risks. This is why experts who care about your health and safety, like the American Academy of Dermatology, stand against *all* forms of body piercing with one exception: the earlobe.

Also, the American Dental Association (ADA) opposes all oral piercing, which includes the tongue, lips, and cheeks. The ADA even calls it a public health hazard. Why? Tongue jewelry can frequently cause chipped or damaged teeth, and it can also cause nasty and dangerous infections.

The U.S. and Canadian Red Cross organizations will not accept a blood donation from someone who's had a body piercing within the last year. Why? Because piercing can spread infections to you (like hepatitis B or C) that can then spread through your blood to others. These infections can harm your liver and even kill you. There is no cure for hepatitis B or C, and the costly treatment of these infections can make you very sick. Who wants that?

The mouth is the area with the most complications from piercings. Besides the general risks, the mouth carries extra dangers:

- Swallowing the jewelry
- Altered eating habits
- Loss of taste
- Injury to your salivary glands

Other problems that are frequently reported include:

- Worn tooth surface
- Damage to your gums and jawline from wear
- Aspiration (inhaling) of a loose piece of jewelry into the lung
- Beaded jewelry becoming trapped between teeth
- Infection and swelling of the tongue

Also, when tongue rings are placed incorrectly, they can cause a nerve problem (*neuropathy*) that really hurts. Some kids who get this say they have shooting pains up to forty times a day. The only thing that helps them is to remove the tongue ring and allow the hole to close up.

So why is it okay to pierce the earlobe? The ear lobe is made of fatty tissue and has a great blood supply. If it gets infected, high levels of infection-fighting cells from the bloodstream protect the earlobe. Still, the equipment used must be sterile and brand new. Although earrings can be sterilized before use, most *reusable* piercing guns are not sterilized between procedures. Ear piercing systems that use disposable sterile cassettes are the safest, and that's what we recommend.

Many types of ear piercings have become popular, especially piercing through the cartilage of the middle to upper ear. Unfortunately, these *high ear piercings* have many more complications than lower earlobe piercings, including poor healing and more serious infections. This is because ear cartilage contains very few of the blood vessels that bring infection-fighting cells to the area pierced.

Cartilage infections in the ear typically occur in the first month after piercing. The significant scarring that can result from these infections may last a lifetime or require plastic surgery to repair.

Body piercings can also have social and emotional consequences. Think about this. How many politicians, business leaders, pastors, physicians, attorneys, judges, and newscasters do you see with exposed piercings? Not very many, right? Why do you think this is?

We think it's because, right or not, people with body piercings are judged. That's just the way it is. Many people make negative value judgments about people with piercings — especially girls and women. We're not saying these judgments are correct. They

A Fierce Pierce

Other risks of having a body part pierced include:

- Infections (especially staph infections) and boils (painful infections under the skin that can lead to ugly scars)
- Nerve damage causing local paralysis, numbness, or lasting pain
- Skin allergies to the jewelry that's used
- Scarring (especially around the lips or eyes)
- Sepsis (a blood infection sometimes called *blood poisoning*)
- Raised, noticeable scars called *keloids*
- Excessive bleeding requiring an expensive emergency room visit
- Permanent holes or deforming scars in your nose or eyebrow
- Chipped or broken teeth (with tongue piercings)
- A speech impediment (while the tongue jewelry is in place)
- Rarely, hepatitis B, hepatitis C, tetanus, or HIV

More than 35 percent of people who get body piercings experience one or more of these problems. So if you're thinking about piercing, ask yourself, is the pierce worth the fears and all the future tears? There's a lot of regret associated with such a small piece of jewelry.

likely are not. But the truth is that such judgmental attitudes could prevent you from getting a job you want down the road. Even if you remove the jewelry, the hole it leaves can be that telltale mark that can be used against you.

So here's the bottom line. Don't think that we're telling you all this stuff to frighten you. We're not. We simply want you to be wise in the decisions you make about your body.

If you are considering a body piercing, we just want you to understand ahead of time that it can lead to lasting problems even if you don't have complications from the piercing. Before you get one, make sure you're prepared for any of the dangers and social consequences that may come with body piercings.

Think long and hard before you get anything other than your ears pierced. You'll usually need a parent's permission and signature anyway, so talk it over with them and pray about it.

If your parents say to wait until you're older, trust that they have good reasons. And if your best friends or that *still, quiet voice* deep inside your soul says wait, trust that advice too.

> Do you not know that your bodies are temples of the Holy Spirit, who is in you, whom you have received from God? You are not your own; you were bought at a price. Therefore honor God with your bodies.
>
> *1 Corinthians 6:19–20*

QUESTION 25

Thinking about inking — are temporary tattoos safe?

Have you been tempted to get a heart, butterfly, or tiny flower tattoo somewhere on your body where most people won't see it? Or do you have friends who already have a tattoo?

If you'd never get a permanent tattoo (which we'll talk about in the next question), have you considered getting a temporary one at a tourist shop or attraction while on vacation?

When we say temporary tattoos, we're not talking about the kind you put on with a wet washcloth. We mean the so-called "temporary" tattoos that are usually made with black henna and are meant to fade over days or weeks.

You're probably wondering what on earth black henna is. No, this has nothing to do with hens or any type of poultry. Henna is a plant that's been used for thousands of years to dye anything from leather to hair, skin, and fingernails.

Since henna can be applied without piercing your skin, it is technically not a tattoo. Tattooing is placing a permanent mark on the skin by inserting pigment or dye *into* or *under* the skin. Though black henna marks are technically not tattoos, they are *not* necessarily safe.

Although henna markings on the skin pose almost no risk of hepatitis, AIDS, or the other serious health risks associated with traditional tattoos, henna markings can cause other problems such as severe allergic reactions, bad skinburns, and even permanent, ugly scarring.

The U.S. Food and Drug Administration (FDA) does *not* approve henna for direct application to the skin. Henna is approved only for use as a hair dye. Its use on a person's skin is illegal, yet henna "tattoos" sure are easy to obtain.

Many parents have filed lawsuits against distributors of black henna after their children were scarred by black henna markings—but the damage has already happened. In each case, neither the girls involved nor their parents knew of the potential danger. But now you do. So you'll be able to warn any of your friends who are considering this type of tattoo.

Although most girls won't experience a problem with henna tattoos, some could be permanently scarred with a forever reminder of their "temporary" poor decision.

> So whether you eat or drink or whatever you do, do it all for the glory of God.
>
> *1 Corinthians 10:31*

QUESTION 26

What about permanent tattoos?

With so many athletes, TV celebrities, and movie stars sporting tattoos these days, you may think it's a cool idea to get one someday. Although tattoos used to be a guy thing, tons of people get tattoos nowadays, including women.

In 1936, *LIFE* magazine estimated that only about 6 percent of people in America had at least one tattoo—and they were mostly men. But by 2012 the American Medical Association (AMA) reported 36 percent of eighteen- to twenty-five-year-olds had a tattoo, and nearly one in five of them were women.

Sadly, most people who get tattooed don't know the health risks. I (Dr. Walt) think that all tattooing should require a signed consent form outlining all the risks—the most obvious one being a major case of remorse. One-half of people who get a tattoo later wish they hadn't. Also, did you know it's illegal for minors to be tattooed in most states? And even within states, the laws can be different from town to town.

So what are some of the risks of getting a tattoo? Tattooing can be very painful. And once done, if you change your mind, tattoos are even more painful (and very expensive) to remove. A tattoo that costs several hundred dollars could require several thousand dollars and many laser sessions to remove. And removing tattoos can leave ugly scars.

And get this! There's no regulation that requires tattoo inks to be sterile (clean and free of infections). Can you believe that? It's true. Worse yet, tattooing can infect you with diseases that make you very sick.

In most states, tattoo parlors are not regulated. Unclean equipment, ink, or technique can infect you with a lifelong, incurable infection — such as HIV (the virus that causes AIDS) or hepatitis B or C (which can harm your liver and cause liver cancer or death). Tattooing can also spread syphilis, tuberculosis, and other diseases from one person to another.

One study reported that the commercial tattoo industry may be the number one distributor of hepatitis C. They found that you are twice as likely to be infected with hepatitis C from getting a tattoo than by shooting up dope (injecting drugs into your veins). That's pretty scary.

Because of the risk of these infections, the American Association of Blood Banks and the Red Cross won't accept blood donations until one year after a person gets a tattoo. They wait a year to see if an infection shows up. They know that if you get a tattoo, you can end up with a two-for-one deal: a forever tattoo with a side order of hepatitis. Not such a happy meal, is it? And if you get a tattoo, there's likely another needle in your future. Your doctor will want blood work to check for this cancer-causing and potentially deadly virus.

More Risks of Having a Tattoo

- Tattooing can cause skin infections, including MRSA, which is tough to treat and can lead to scarring.

- Even tattoo artists who use clean tools and technique have clients who have been infected with a germ similar to the one that causes tuberculosis.

- Some unlicensed tattoo artists use printer ink rather than tattoo ink and guitar strings instead of needles (no, that doesn't mean your tattoo will sing). Do you think that's all clean and infection-free? *No way!*

- Bumps called *granulomas* can form around tattoo ink — especially red ink.

- Tattooing can lead to a keloid, a scar that gets very thick and raised.

- Since some of the dyes used are not approved for use in people, your skin can stay irritated for years.

- Although rare, some people have allergic reactions to the pigments. These reactions can be severe and cause terrible ulcers or scarring. We've seen patients with severe scarring from both tattooing and tattoo removal.

While we were writing this book, a mysterious outbreak of nasty skin rashes in upstate New York was traced to contaminated water in tattoo ink.

An Unusual Tattoo

Years ago, I (Dr. Mari) saw such an interesting tattoo, I had to ask about it. While doing a physical exam on a college student, I noticed a black vertical line above her nipple. When I asked her why she had a line on her breast, she sighed.

"It used to be a small butterfly," she recalled, "but after I gained weight, my breasts grew, and the tattoo stretched out too. So now I have a line above my breast. Who wants that?"

Then she added, "Please tell other girls to think twice before they do something like this. You never know how things will change."

Many tattoo inks contain an unknown mixture of chemicals. Many of these chemicals were intended for use in writing and printer inks as well as car paint—but never for use in or under the skin. It is impossible to know for sure what's in tattoo ink. There's also concern that some ingredients in tattoo ink may contribute to or cause cancer.

By far the most common "side effect" of a tattoo is regret. We can't count the number of people we've cared for who wish they had thought twice before getting a tattoo. We've even seen people who wanted their tattoos removed within a week of getting them.

Researchers at Texas Tech University report some reasons why people change their minds about tattoos. These include problems wearing clothes, embarrassment, and concerns that tattoos could adversely affect their job or career.

Most people who want to get rid of a tattoo are women. Studies show they feel more judged, like they've been marked with

Are Tattoos Okay for Christians?

Dr. Linda Mintle, a licensed marriage and family therapist and expert on family issues, writes:

> Christians need to consider their motivation for wanting a tattoo.
>
> If the motivation to get a tattoo is to conform to this world and fit in better, bring attention to self versus glorify God, disobey parents and cause the people around them to stumble, then it is not a good idea.
>
> For those who are radically saved and new in Christ, the motivation may be to witness to those who are lost. The bottom line is you have to judge your heart against the Word. God knows your heart and your motives, so an appraisal of motivation is needed.

more than the heart or pony or whatever design they chose. They sense that having a tattoo affects how others see them, which affects how they feel about themselves.

To remove a tattoo, a person often needs ten or more laser treatments several weeks apart. Experts say the average tattoo costs $2,000 to $3,000 to remove. Sadly, after spending all that money, one in four people cannot have their tattoo successfully removed.

So what's the bottom line? Never get a tattoo without giving yourself time (weeks, months, or even years) to think and pray about it. Listen to your parents and never get an illegal tattoo. Double-check your motives for getting a tattoo with someone you admire and trust. And remember that permanent probably means forever, and temporary might too.

Perhaps the most important question is the one that one of our teen reviewers recommends we each ask: "Am I considering doing this for God's glory, or my glory?" Great question.

> And you also were included in Christ when you heard the message of truth, the gospel of your salvation. When you believed, you were marked in him with a seal, the promised Holy Spirit.
>
> *Ephesians 1:13*

Before Getting a Tattoo, Ask Yourself ...

- Why do I want a tattoo?
- Does my motivation to get a tattoo line up with what the Bible teaches?
- What are my heart and conscience saying to me?
- Is the Holy Spirit telling me to do this or encouraging me not to?
- Am I 100 percent sure I'll still want this tattoo or piercing years from now?
- What might my future husband think about this?
- Am I willing to give up potential educational or job opportunities for this tattoo?
- Will I cause a weaker sister or brother to stumble if I get a tattoo?

QUESTION 27

Why are some girls so mean?

Imagine you're at lunch when your friends start making fun of a shy girl who's new to the school. She's sitting all alone, with a near-empty tray of food and a blank stare.

Will you laugh at your friends' comments about her clothes and hair, or will you go sit next to her and help her feel more comfortable?

It's your choice. It's *always* your choice.

If you want to do what's right but worry about what your friends will say or think, you're experiencing peer pressure. A peer is someone your age who is affected by similar stresses and challenges as you. Everyone has peers, regardless of their age. And everyone experiences *peer pressure*—the pressure to fit in or to go along with the crowd. Peer pressure can make you compromise your values and beliefs simply to get a laugh from your "group" or so they will continue to "like" and "accept" you.

The Bible is clear that the wrong kind of peer pressure can keep you from God's best:

> Do not follow the crowd in doing wrong.
>
> *Exodus 23:2*

> And so I insist—and God backs me up on this—that there be no going along with the crowd, the empty-headed, mindless crowd. They've refused for so long to deal with God that they've lost touch not only with God but with reality itself. They can't think straight anymore.
>
> *Ephesians 4:17–18 MSG*

Part of maturing means learning to make wise choices consistently. That means you make good, healthy, and smart choices based on God's plans for your life. But even though girls' brains mature at a young age, they don't always behave like it. You may have experienced this at school or in your neighborhood. Sometimes girls are just plain mean. These girls don't always choose to be nice or *act* maturely even if their brain is capable of it.

Still, *you* can choose to be kind to the new girl in school even if it feels uncomfortable. You can choose to be different. You can decide to be yourself, even if it means that your "friends" won't accept you.

And here's the truth about that. If you need to change who you are so that others like and accept you, they are not true friends.

You can choose to do what's right—which may often be the hardest of the choices you'll have. And, yes, some people might make fun of you, but your heart will be at peace knowing you did the right thing. And who knows? Maybe you'll make a new friend for life.

How to Keep Your Cool

You may experience the same emotions as a mean bully, but you can choose not to behave in angry ways that hurt others. So what can you do when you're angry?

- *You can* take a deep breath and count to ten.
- *You can* walk away from the situation.
- *You can* find someone to talk to, like a parent, your sister, or a good friend.
- *You can* do something active like jogging or biking — great ways to burn off steam.
- *You can* pray and recall scriptures that help you remember who you are and God's best for you.
- *You can* choose not to be mean or hurtful to others or to yourself.
- *You can* choose to be kind when it would be easier to offend or insult others.
- *You can* think of something you love to do and add it to this list!

So, you see, there is much *you can* do when you're angry. Just don't stay angry. That's not good for anyone, especially you.

Even if you make good choices, the reality is that some people choose to be mean and even enjoy bullying others. But bullying is not God's plan for anyone. God never wants us to be mean to others.

Boys tend to be mean by hitting, pushing, or being physical, while girls are often mean in more verbal and relational ways, such as through insults or ignoring. Boys tend to intimidate through their strength or physical attributes. Girls often hurt others emotionally by excluding, teasing, and mocking. Ouch.

None of this is good for anyone, but it happens a lot. You may see it more during the tween and teen years. It helps to know what's happening, and understanding will help you know how to respond.

So what's the difference between meanness and just being moody, which we all experience at times? In question 17 we addressed moodiness as a normal part of growing up that can be managed in various ways. Moods are one thing; meanness is quite another. Moods are usually short-lived, whereas meanness can become a habit, even a way of life. Moods come upon us unexpectedly, but meanness is a choice.

We all go through tough times, and we all have bad moods or sad days. We all feel angry at times, but we don't have to act out in sadness or anger toward others. As with moodiness, we can learn to manage how we *feel* and choose to act upon what we *know* instead.

"In your anger do not sin": Do not let the sun go down while you are still angry, and do not give the devil a foothold.

Ephesians 4:26–27

God gave us our emotions, but he also gave us the ability to make good and wise choices. Although at times we will be angry, confused, and frustrated, we must avoid sinning because of how we *feel*. If we stay angry, this Scripture passage says we give the devil a foothold. What happens if someone grabs your foot? You trip, right? And land flat on your face.

Staying angry is like opening a faucet so that water keeps gushing out. Until we shut off the faucet of anger, it can lead to more angry actions. It gets easier to sin when tempted because our emotions are out of control. Letting bad feelings control what we do can turn meanness into bullying or violence if we're not careful. So we need to shut off that faucet for good.

Still, not every girl makes these wise choices. Perhaps no one taught her how to be nice to others. Maybe someone yells at her at home and she takes it out on others at school when no adult

Dealing with a Bully

- Do not give in to a bully's demands. Remember: they want to control you by shocking you, upsetting you, and putting you down. Stand up tall, and tell them to stop.

- If they don't stop, keep cool and walk away. When bullies come upon that kind of boldness, they will usually find someone else to pick on.

- If you get an email, text, or instant message that's mean or hurtful (cyber bullying), or if someone posts inappropriate pictures of you or lies about you, tell your parents and/or teacher immediately. This is not acceptable, ever, and must stop.

- Choose friends who are not rude, abusive, or offensive. Don't spend your time with people who enjoy gossiping, being mean to others, or criticizing. Pray for them, but invest your precious time with someone else — someone who really cares about you. Someone who builds you up and encourages you rather than insults you.

- Although a bully's mean behavior may be a cry for help, what he or she is doing is wrong and needs to be handled by an adult. Many bullies need help from a counselor or therapist with special training.

is watching. Sadly, this is the situation for many bullies. They may mistreat others because they're hurting inside, and that's how they've learned to behave.

Some girls use technology to be mean to other girls. It's called *cyber bullying*. Although we know you've heard of this and may have been exposed to it already, let's define some terms so we're all on the same page.

A bully is someone who continually picks on someone else, usually another kid who is smaller, shy, or insecure. Bullies love to get a response; they feel powerful if they can control someone else by demeaning, insulting, or just being mean.

Although bullying in person is more common for boys, girls are more likely to cyber bully. They send emails, instant messages, or texts loaded with hurtful words they wouldn't dare say in person—but will say behind the "safe" cover of technology.

A new form of bullying is called *burning*—what we call *bullying on steroids*. This is a cruel game where everything someone says is turned upside down and distorted into a joke. Girl bullies write "burn books" packed with hurtful lies about a girl, spreading rumors or making fun of the way she looks or who she is.

Typically, a cyber bully singles out someone, opens an Internet page in that person's name, and posts gross and hurtful lies about her. This is wrong and illegal. Social media sites and schools have worked together with police officers to take down these burn pages. Those responsible face possible criminal charges and can even be thrown in jail.

Beyond these types of bullying, some girls seem to enjoy putting other girls down by gossiping about them. Gossip, while not the same as bullying, is another dangerous and hurtful practice that, for some girls, becomes a way of life. Through gossip, these girls criticize or make fun of the way other girls look, talk, dress, or behave—pretty much anything. We like this saying: *Gossip* is saying behind someone's back what you wouldn't say to their face, while *flattery* is saying to someone's face what you wouldn't say behind their back. Both are wrong.

Did you know that the Bible speaks about the destructive power of gossip?

> Avoid godless chatter, because those who indulge in it will become more and more ungodly.
>
> *2 Timothy 2:16*

Though some tongues just love the taste of gossip, those who follow Jesus have better uses for language than that. Don't talk dirty or silly. That kind of talk doesn't fit our style. Thanksgiving is our dialect.

Ephesians 5:3–4 MSG

Mean people spread mean gossip; their words smart and burn.

Proverbs 16:27 MSG

Listening to gossip is like eating cheap candy; do you want junk like that in your belly?

Proverbs 26:22 MSG

So what can you do when girls are mean through gossip?

Start by avoiding these types of conversations. If someone gossips, don't throw more wood in that fire. Instead, get in the habit of saying something like, "I prefer not to talk about that because I don't know if it's true," and change the subject. That's a great way to extinguish the spreading flames of gossip.

If they don't stop after a minute, you can say, "Okay, okay. Can we talk about something else now?" Or you can be more direct and say, "I don't like gossip. Please stop talking like this."

Or you could ask, "Would you say that to the face of the person you're talking about?" Usually, they wouldn't.

As you do this more and more, your friends will recognize that you don't like gossip. You may even help them rethink what they are talking about.

An important way to deal with meanness is by choosing your friends well. Is a girl nice to you one day and mean the next? Does she talk about others all the time? Does she criticize you or make you feel bad about yourself? If so, ask yourself, *Is this a girl I really want to hang out with?*

If you're involved in a conflict with a friend, try talking about your feelings. Take your friend aside, and just between the two of you, say:

- "It hurts my feelings when you say these things about me."
- "It made me feel bad when you made fun of my [clothes, hair, etc.]."
- "I had asked you not to say anything about that, and I'm really mad that you did."

A true friend won't be angry with you for saying something. Or she may be upset at first but then apologize later. It takes courage to be honest, but every time you speak the truth, you'll feel better inside. You may also help others when you take a stand for what is right and speak up.

If you and a friend get into a fight, or the rumor mill spreads something untrue, don't let your anger linger. Go to your friend right away and set the record straight.

- "Did you really say that about me?"
- "I'm sorry. I didn't mean to hurt your feelings."
- "Your friendship means so much to me. Can we talk about what happened?"

If you wait, your mind may make the problem into something bigger. You can start to imagine things that are untrue, and pretty soon you feel worse and worse. Don't hesitate. Make things right as soon as possible. Pray for the words. Pray for wisdom. Though conflict is hard, every time you take a brave step, you will grow stronger in your faith. And it will be easier the next time something happens.

> "Therefore, if you are offering your gift at the altar and there remember that your brother or sister has something against you, leave your gift there in front of the altar. First go and be reconciled to them; then come and offer your gift."
>
> *Matthew 5:23–24*

The Making of a Good Friend

What makes a good friend? Here's how my (Dr. Mari's) son recently described his best friend. "He makes it easy, Mom. I never have to worry about what I say or do. I can just be myself. He accepts me just the way I am."

He's right. Being with a good friend makes you feel good, not stressed. A good friend doesn't try to change you in order to love and accept you, but he or she challenges you to be your very best every day.

I've had three "best friends" since middle school. We are true BFFs. We're all different. Two are teachers, one's a musician, and I'm a doctor and writer. We also have many things in common. These are some of the things that have made us great lifelong friends:

- We love, encourage, and help each other.
- We tell the truth, especially when it's hard.
- We stand by one another in good times and bad.
- We've shared important life experiences, like going to school and serving others.
- Our families know and trust each other; we are close to our parents and to one another.
- When going through tough times, like when my parents split up, we always help each other.
- While in school, we always looked out for one another at parties.
- Now, as adults, we stay close even while living miles apart.

Some girls are mean, but thankfully, most girls are not. Good friends are one of the best things in life.

A friend loves at all times.

Proverbs 17:17

If you or a friend continues to be bullied despite your best efforts, tell a teacher or school counselor and discuss it with your parents. Don't keep it to yourself. Tell your parents or guardians what's going on so they can help you. If you'd prefer, your mom or dad can talk to your teacher. And if your parents can't or won't help, consider asking another trusted adult (like a teacher, school principal, or coach).

Remember, if it's happening to you, it is probably happening to others in your school. Stopping abusive behavior will help many people, including you, your friends, and even bullies.

So why are some girls so mean? Because they choose to be. But *you* don't have to. Surround yourself with people who love and respect you, and remember to pray for those who don't.

> Make sure that nobody pays back wrong for wrong, but always strive to do what is good for each other and for everyone else.
>
> *1 Thessalonians 5:15*

> Whoever of you loves life and desires to see many good days, keep your tongue from evil and your lips from telling lies. Turn from evil and do good; seek peace and pursue it.
>
> *Psalm 34:12–14*

> Be kind and compassionate to one another, forgiving each other, just as in Christ God forgave you.
>
> *Ephesians 4:32*

> Likewise, the tongue is a small part of the body, but it makes great boasts. Consider what a great forest is set on fire by a small spark.
>
> *James 3:5*

QUESTION 28

Social media is fun, but how much is too much?

Can you imagine life with no Internet? No mp3 players, no texting? No iPods or TV? None of this was around when we (and your parents) were kids, but now they're in every home and pocket—including yours, right?

Today's technology is mind-boggling. The Internet connects us with the world like never before. Families and friends keep in touch through social media: Skype, Facebook, Twitter, Pinterest, Face Time, Google Plus, online gaming, Instagram.

All this technology can be great, but when can it become harmful?

It's critical to understand that the Internet is potentially dangerous. It brings good and bad into your life, including things you may not otherwise look at. Sexy images and even people with bad intentions are as real and up close as your next email, IM, or pop-up.

So how can you make the most of the Internet and social media while avoiding the bad?

Here's a great starting point. Never post anything online, in an IM, email, or social media site, that you wouldn't say or do in person — or that you wouldn't want printed in the school newspaper or yearbook!

Before you post anything at all, ask yourself, *Would I say this to someone face-to-face? Will I be proud if the word gets out that I posted this?*

Ask yourself these questions when using social media:

1. What does this text or photo say about what I value and about me?
2. How might this text or photo impact those who see it?
3. Does this post, text, or photo bring glory to God?

These questions will serve as a wise filter to help you do the right thing while using technology. Even pictures of people in bathing suits posted on social media can cross a line pretty quickly. Remember, if what you post doesn't show that you respect yourself, and if you don't protect your dignity as God's child, will others?

We like the saying, "Everything speaks." Everything you see, hear, and read conveys a message. And *everything* that goes online, whether in an email or a text, stays there *forever* — and can become public at any time in your life. So think twice before you post, text, or write anything at all.

The average teen sends 3,339 texts per month. That's about 110 per day and climbing. Texting can take over your life if you're not careful.

Since girls value communication and connection so much, texting and social media can get out of hand very quickly. Sadly,

WWJTXT?

There is now a *What Would Jesus Text?* movement among tweens, teens, and young adults. A thumb ring reminds you to think before you text. The ministry, which you can find with this QR code or the URL in our list of resources, is based on this verse:

What Would Jesus Text?

> May these words of my mouth and this meditation of my heart be pleasing in your sight, LORD, my Rock and my Redeemer.
>
> Psalm 19:14

Here's the message that comes with each thumb band:

> When texting, we are sometimes faced with temptations that can be hard to overcome. Because we're human and not perfect, we sometimes make mistakes. Let this thumb band be a gentle reminder to do what's right. Ask yourself, "What would Jesus text?" So, when you look back at the end of the day, you'll have no regrets.

You can also write a scripture like Psalm 19:14 or a note on your computer, tablet, iPod, and phone to remind you to be wise in all things, including social media.

research has found that girls who spend a lot of time on social media (like Facebook or Twitter) tend to dislike their bodies and themselves more. They are also more likely to have depression and lower self-esteem. This is not surprising, since the media in general—including social media—is obsessed with the wrong kind of beauty (as you learned in question 9).

Girls who overuse social media get extra doses of the lie that skinnier and sexier is better. Then when they look in the mirror and don't see a skinny-sexy-photoshopped model, they may begin to feel discouraged, even depressed. This makes perfect sense. Research shows that the more screen time for girls, the less happy they are with their weight and body image, and the more obsessed they are with thinness and outer appearance.

So don't overdo it with social media and the Internet. These are great tools to use for learning and connecting with friends and family, but they can harm you as well. Be careful and use limits, like spending no more than thirty minutes to an hour a day online (or less).

So what else can you do to protect yourself from the dangers of social media and the Internet?

- Keep all electronics outside your bedroom. Have one room in the main part of the house for all electronics: smartphones, mp3 players, tablets, and computers. This will keep the whole family more accountable.
- When you get home, don't keep your phone and iPod in your pocket. Park them in the computer room. This way, when Patty and Susie text you three times in a row to plan the next movie night, you're not tempted to answer immediately while ignoring your family or your studies. You'll enjoy people more if you stay focused on them.
- Discuss with your parents when to turn everything off. Consider these guidelines:

   Tweens: No video games, social media, or Internet (apart from homework) after 6:00 p.m., and none unless you've been physically active and/or played outside for a while—which is fun and so good for you.

   Teens: Phones, computers, and all electronics go off no later than 9:00 p.m. on weeknights. No texting after 9:00 p.m. on school nights, possibly a bit later on weekends. All electronics sleep in the "off" position in the designated family computer room—not in your bedroom.

Text, Sext — What's Next?

Sexting is sending sexually explicit messages or photos, usually between cell phones. One study found that nearly 40 percent of tweens and teens have received an "offensive or distressing" sexual image by text or email.

Not only is it illegal to send or store a sext of a minor, it's also wrong, unwise, and potentially dangerous. Some teens who have sexted photographs of themselves, or of their friends, have been charged with spreading child pornography. And others, who have received the images, have been charged with possession of child pornography. These are both crimes.

Many states have laws requiring mandatory sentencing of *anyone* who has photos like that of someone under sixteen, even if they didn't ask for it to be sent to them. The bottom line is that if it's found on your phone or computer, you are breaking the law and could end up in trouble with the cops. Do yourself a favor and avoid that at all costs.

All ages: No access to video games, TV, social media, texts, or email until all homework is complete unless a parent makes an exception.

You can ask your parents if these guidelines can be relaxed as rewards for good behavior, on special occasions, and on weekends. And remember these tips:

- Don't overdo it with technology. It's not good for you or your relationships.
- Be considerate. Sitting in front of someone at the dinner table while texting away is rude. It sends the message that

the person you're texting is more important than the person in front of you. Stay present with the people around you.

• Respect your siblings, parents, teachers, and friends. If they're in front of you, give them your full attention.

Remember, once a text, email, or sext is on the Internet, it's *always* on the Internet. It cannot be erased. And *any* sext, no matter who sends it, can end up on a porn site. The Internet Watch Foundation estimates that nearly 90 percent of sexts were stolen from their original upload location (typically social networks) and posted on other websites—especially porn sites that collect inappropriate images of children and young people.

Imagine anything you write or any picture you send being seen by your parents, your friends, your pastor, or your priest. What would it be like if your future husband or your future children saw a sext of you? You'd *never* want them to see something embarrassing or inappropriate you posted, would you? Then don't do it.

Believe it or not, we've even heard of kids who didn't get into college or didn't get a job they really wanted because of this. Why? Because colleges and employers routinely Google those who apply to their schools and jobs. Anything inappropriate they find can be used against you, even a picture posted as a joke. They also search social media sites like Facebook to try to find out more about you. So be smart, and do the right thing.

If someone asks you to sext, tell your parents or a trusted adult immediately and unfriend or block posts or texts from this person. Avoid sexting at all costs—sending *and* receiving. If you get a sext or inappropriate message, tell your parent or teacher, a counselor, or a trusted adult. Don't let it go on.

Another great idea is to have electronics-free weekends and screen-free breaks to rest your mind and focus on other things. This may sound awful, but you'll thank us.

How Many Ways Can You Say No?

Recently I (Dr. Walt) heard an ad from the Ad Council on the radio where a preteen tested different ways to say no if someone asks her for a sext. We added some of our own one-liners to her clever list. Can you think of any others?

- No way, José!
- I'm camera shy.
- I already said no.
- It's against my religion.
- I'm giving my dog a bath, you can have pictures of that.
- Pressure gives me hives.
- Under my clothes I'm a robot.
- Hold on; let me ask my mom.
- Sorry, a horse ate my webcam.
- I'm worried they'll get passed around school.
- Unfortunately I just had my clothes surgically attached to my body.
- If they got out I might never be president.
- Not even if you were all three Jonas Brothers.
- I have a rash.
- I have lizard skin.
- The more you ask, the uglier you get.
- Is there a bug in your ear?
- You're not the boss of me.
- Did you forget I said no?

The ad ends by saying, "When someone is pressuring you to do something you don't want to do, how many ways can you say no before they get the message?" Can you and your friends come up with more ways to just say no?

Sexting Invaded My Home

One of our reviewers shared this personal story:

My parents gave me a cell phone for safety reasons when I went to middle school. We all were very naive and didn't think about having some guidelines to go along with it.

My parents never read the texts that were coming in or going out. They also didn't realize that I should have time restraints with phone use. This caused me to have less sleep as well, staying up late to answer the texts of my night-owl friends.

Without my parents knowing it, a boy in my school began sexting me. It was both gross and embarrassing — especially since I only wanted a good relationship with him. But because my parents and I didn't have any ground rules, clear expectations, clear communications, or an open-phone policy, I was scared to tell my parents about it.

The sexts kept coming and caused me a great deal of confusion and heartache. I didn't know what to do, until the communication with him was suddenly blocked. How? Thank goodness my parents finally figured out what was going on and put a stop to it.

It would have been so much easier to stop things before they started if my parents and I had only been on the same page. By sharing my experience with other girls my age, I hope to spare others some of the pain our family encountered.

So when your parents read your texts, know that they're trying to protect you.

Go outside. Take walks without being tied to a cell phone or iPod. Breathe in some fresh air. Ride your bike. Write a letter to a friend or to a grandparent, aunt, or cousin. Send a card to someone serving in the military. Read a good book, or visit your local library. Do a puzzle, or paint something. Visit someone at a nursing home. Volunteer to serve food at a homeless shelter or soup kitchen. Work at a food pantry. Find a new hobby. Just stand on your head—anything. You may discover a new talent if you turn off the TV, shut down your computer, and put away your phone. Give it a try.

And speaking of good books to read and movies to watch, be selective. What you read and watch feeds your mind, your heart, and your soul. Be wise, and choose well. Some books and movies that are promoted to young girls shouldn't even be read or watched by adults.

Ask your parents or other trusted Christian adults before deciding on a book or movie that someone recommends. Before you read something, ask yourself if it will be informative or entertaining in a way that helps or harms you. If you're not sure, find something better to do.

> Do not conform to the pattern of this world, but be transformed by the renewing of your mind. Then you will be able to test and approve what God's will is—his good, pleasing and perfect will.
>
> *Romans 12:2*

> May God himself, the God of peace, sanctify you through and through. May your whole spirit, soul and body be kept blameless at the coming of our Lord Jesus Christ.
>
> *1 Thessalonians 5:23*

Plugged In

Have you ever seen a movie preview and thought, *That looks like a really cool movie?* Then you go see it and it's not at all what you expected. It's boring, scary, or totally inappropriate. If you use resources like Plugged In, you won't ever have that happen again.

Both of our families like Plugged In, a website that analyzes and rates movies, videos, music, TV, and games. You can trust the reviewers to give a thumbs-up or a thumbs-down to media you're thinking of listening to, watching, or reading. They also have a really cool blog and weekly podcast that will keep you and your friends in the know about media.

A typical Plugged In review will assess a movie's:

- Positive elements
- Spiritual, sexual, and violent content
- Drug and alcohol content
- Crude language
- Other negative elements

Next time a friend invites you over for a movie, remember to "plug in" before you buy in. You can find Plugged In with the URL in our resources list at the back of the book.

QUESTION 29

What if my friends want to try alcohol, drugs, or dangerous games?

In question 26 we mentioned that many people regret getting a tattoo within a week of getting it. Some regret it the next day. You know why? Because they were drunk, stoned, or high on drugs when they got it.

Imagine waking up one morning, looking down your arm, and doing a double take. Shocked, you realize the lizard you just spotted there will now walk with you everywhere — 'cause it's tattooed on your arm. That's the kind of stuff people sometimes do when they drink or use drugs. Not such a great idea, is it?

You may not feel tempted to drink alcohol, but some kids you know are likely already drinking or talking about it. Sadly, nearly one in four girls starts drinking alcohol before age thirteen.

A lot of girls we talk to don't know that alcohol in all forms

193

(wine, beer, and liquor) is a drug—an illegal drug if you're under twenty-one years of age. So for followers of Jesus, underage drinking is a sin because it breaks the law. For a lot of girls, this is enough to help them decide alcohol isn't worth the trouble.

Did you know it's easier to get hooked on alcohol or other drugs when you're younger? This means you want more and more of it each day; you're *addicted*. People who get hooked on alcohol or drugs make very poor choices, like stealing or hurting others to get money to pay for more booze or drugs. So one sin leads to another and another. It's a terrible cycle that's best to avoid completely.

Girls who drink before age fifteen are five times more likely to have problems with alcohol later in life. So if you or your friends start drinking at your age, you are much more likely to get hooked on alcohol even as a teen.

Addiction to alcohol is known as *alcoholism*, and people with this addiction are called *alcoholics*. Being hooked on alcohol (or drugs) traps you in a prison of sorts—physically, emotionally, relationally, and spiritually. Using drugs affects *everything* about you. The good news is that this is totally preventable, especially when you realize that most alcoholics begin drinking when they are very young. So don't.

Drinking even small amounts of alcohol affects girls differently than boys. Girls are much more sensitive to the effects of alcohol than boys, so it is much more dangerous for women than it is for men. Did you know that? More female alcoholics die from suicide, alcohol-related injuries, circulatory disorders, and a bad liver disease called *cirrhosis* than male alcoholics.

Having even one drink per day increases the risk of at least eight types of cancer (mouth, pharynx, larynx, esophagus, liver, breast, colon, and rectum) and many other serious conditions (such as seizure disorders, inflammation of the pancreas [a digestive gland], stroke, heartbeat irregularities, cirrhosis, and high blood pressure).

Did You Know?

The National Center on Addiction and Substance Abuse at Columbia University published some interesting facts about girls and substance abuse:

SMOKING

- Nearly one in every four high school senior girls smokes.
- Girls get hooked on cigarettes quicker than boys.
- Many teens who take birth control pills also smoke. Taken together, cigarettes and the pill can cause heart problems and dangerous blood clots.

ALCOHOL

- Nearly half of high school girls drink alcohol.
- Nearly one in four girls starts drinking before age thirteen.
- Drinking before age fifteen quadruples the chances of getting hooked on alcohol.
- Teen girls who drink a lot are way more likely to have sex (particularly unwanted sex) than girls who don't drink.
- Compared to boys, girls get drunk faster, get hooked on alcohol more quickly, and develop heart, liver, and brain problems sooner.
- For girls, one drink usually has the same effect as two to three drinks for a boy.
- Teen girls who drink often are almost six times more likely to attempt suicide than girls who never drink.

OTHER DRUGS

- Girls who smoke marijuana have more suicidal thoughts and suicide attempts than girls who don't.
- Painkillers are the most abused prescription drugs among teen girls.
- Teen girls are more likely than boys to use over-the-counter drugs to get high. And these medicines can be just as dangerous as prescription drugs.

For females, including teens, even one drink a day increases the risk for breast cancer. Women who have three or more drinks a week have a 15 percent higher risk of breast cancer. And the chances go up even more for each additional drink women regularly have each day. So for girls and women, when it comes to cancer prevention, there's no amount of alcohol that can be said to be safe.

The bottom line is that drinking alcohol can harm your health. So be smart and choose to say no to alcohol and all illegal drugs.

Pot's the Pits

Teens in Colorado, where recreational marijuana (pot) use is now legal for adults, believe these lies about it:

- They think pot actually helps brain cells grow and develop.
- They know smoking pot is bad for your lungs, but they think it's safer than smoking cigarettes.
- They think pot helps you focus in class.

But *none* of these beliefs is true. Here are the facts and just a few of the reasons we tell teens (and everyone) to avoid marijuana:

- Marijuana, also known as *pot*, *weed*, or *joints*, is a drug.
- Marijuana is bad for you, your brain, and your life.
- Teens make bad decisions when they smoke pot, including:
  —Driving and wrecking a car — potentially killing themselves or someone else.
  —Making sexual choices that are unsafe or out of character.
  —Saying or doing dumb or hurtful things they later regret.

The Bible teaches that, as Christians, we are to be wise and cautious in the way we live. We are not to be foolish, and we are not to get drunk:

> Be very careful, then, how you live—not as unwise but as wise.... Therefore do not be foolish, but understand what the Lord's will is. Do not get drunk on wine, which leads to debauchery. Instead, be filled with the Spirit.
>
> *Ephesians 5:15, 17–18*

- Marijuana can also affect your judgment about other drugs. While high on pot, you may drink too much or use drugs you never even planned to try.
- Pot affects your memory and your ability to solve problems. It can also contribute to depression and anxiety, and it can mess up your periods.
- Teens who use marijuana are almost twice as likely to exhibit psychotic behaviors (like seeing or hearing things that aren't real) compared to those who don't.
- Marijuana cigarettes have no filters and contain more tar than nicotine cigarettes. They are even *worse* for your lungs than regular cigarettes (which are bad enough).
- Long-term marijuana use can lead to lung problems like infections, trouble breathing, and cancer.
- Teens are much more likely than adults to get hooked on pot.
- Teens who use pot more than once a week can lower their IQ (a measure of intelligence) for life. In other words, smoking pot can make you dumber. Like one of our teen reviewers said, "No wonder they call it dope."

To be *filled with the Spirit* means to be controlled by, guided by, and empowered by God's Spirit—led by God, not by selfishness. It means to be in control, not out of control.

> You are all children of the light and children of the day. We do not belong to the night or to the darkness. So then, let us not be like others, who are asleep, but let us be awake and sober. For those who sleep, sleep at night, and those who get drunk, get drunk at night. But since we belong to the day, let us be sober, putting on faith and love as a breastplate, and the hope of salvation as a helmet.
>
> *1 Thessalonians 5:5–8*

Here are some of the lies about drugs that you may hear from other kids (and the lies apply to alcohol, marijuana, other inhaled or puffed drugs, and any other drug not prescribed for you):

Lie No. 1: "Drugs will help you deal with your problems."

The truth is, many people use a drug to "numb" their pain. They use it to escape from problems or to forget their troubles. But guess what! When the drug effect wears off, their problems are still there. And now they have even more problems caused by the drug use itself, like wrecking their car or fighting with their best friend. Drugs will never, ever help you solve what is wrong with your life. Drugs will only make things worse.

Lie No. 2: "Drugs will make you look cool."

The truth is, people who drink or use drugs do incredibly uncool things—like stumbling or falling, slurring their speech, having accidents, saying things that hurt others, vomiting their guts out, losing control of their behavior, and many other stupid things.

Worse yet, girls who drink or use drugs and drive end up killing or hurting themselves or others almost every day. Each year, thousands of fifteen- to twenty-year-old drivers are killed in drug-related car accidents, while nearly 300,000 are injured. That's not cool at all.

Lie No. 3: "Drugs will make you happy and help you have a good time."

No doubt about it, drinking alcohol or taking drugs can give you a "buzz" — especially when the drug first begins to affect your brain. And it's not just your brain that's drunk or drugged, but also your entire nervous system. But alcohol and other drugs *never* make a person happy. Alcohol is a depressant. It eventually makes most people feel down and drowsy. It makes them move and react much more slowly than normal.

At first, someone who's drinking alcohol or doing drugs might seem to lose their inhibitions. They "loosen up" and do or say things they normally wouldn't. This is why some people seem wild or out of control when they drink or do drugs. But even if someone seems "pumped up" when they drink, the drug ends up making them sluggish, slow, and unable to make wise decisions.

Experts who work with adolescent sex offenders who were drinking or on drugs often hear the perpetrator say, "It was the alcohol," or "It was the drugs." But these experts say the drug does not make a person do something they don't want to do. The drug makes it easier for a person to cross the boundaries of what they know is right and wrong. You are less likely to think of the consequences of doing something when you are drinking or high on other illegal drugs.

Lie No. 4: "If you just use a little of these drugs, you won't become addicted."

Totally false.

Some kids believe drinking wine or beer is safer than hard alcohol (like whiskey or vodka). The fact is, beer, wine, and hard liquor all contain the exact same drug: alcohol! Also, some kids think trying someone else's prescription drug or smoking a little marijuana won't hurt. But it does.

Many girls we've cared for say they tried alcohol or drugs because their friends were doing it. Peer pressure can be overwhelming—and not just to drink alcohol, but to use or take any drug that is not prescribed for you by your doctor.

In school and in the neighborhood, in clubs and on teams—even in church youth group—you will feel peer pressure to do wrong things. But it's never right to do what's wrong, is it?

There are always consequences for doing wrong things—there's always a price to pay. And sometimes that price can be very, very high.

Think about it. If you are tempted to drink or take another drug because your friends are pushing you to, then it's time to ask a very important question: What would happen if you told them you're not interested in alcohol or drugs?

Would your friends not want to hang out with you anymore because of your decision? If so, were they true friends in the first place?

Of course not. A real friend, a true friend, will respect your decisions, and she won't try to force you into things that are bad for you. Think twice about hanging out with that "friend" anymore. If she's pushing you to try drugs, she hasn't learned how to be a good friend.

Here are some more tips for handling the pressure to try dangerous games, alcohol, or illegal drugs:

- You don't have to do *anything* that you don't want to do.
- You should not do *anything* that is not right to do.
- Giving in to peer pressure never solves problems, but it often *creates* problems.
- Giving in to peer pressure will *not* make people like and respect you more—even if they act like it. Most people actually respect those who stand up for what they believe.

The Choking "Game" — Breathe or Die

As I (Dr. Walt) was writing this chapter, I read a sad headline in our local paper: "A Colorado Springs ninth grader died as a result of playing the 'choking game,' making him the second student to die after playing the game in the last three years."

I remember playing this "game" with friends when I was in elementary school. But this is no game, and no one warned us of its dangers. No one told us that we could die! Sadly, most of the kids who have died playing the "choking game" were eleven to sixteen years old.

So how is this deadly "game" played, and why? Kids do it to get a brief "high." They either choke each other or use a noose or rope to choke themselves. It's crazy! A kid can pass out from this in seconds, get seriously hurt, and even die.

Anything that blocks the arteries in the neck that bring oxygen to the brain will make you pass out. Within three minutes, memory, balance, and other brain functions start to fail. Death occurs shortly after. The choking game has also been called the *pass-out game*, the *strangling game*, *space monkey* or *space cowboy*, *suffocation roulette*, the *fainting game*, *blackout*, *flatliner*, *California choke*, *purple dragon*, or *cloud nine*.

Don't ever play any of these so-called "games." Be smart, and stay safe! You can learn more about the dangers of this game from this QR code or the URL in our resources list at the back of the book.

The Dangers of the Choking Game

With each temptation that comes our way, God provides a way of escape:

> No temptation has overtaken you except what is common to mankind. And God is faithful; he will not let you be tempted beyond what you can bear. But when you are tempted, he will also provide a way out so that you can endure it.

1 Corinthians 10:13

You may wonder, *How can I escape the temptation—the pressure?* Remember, it's always okay to just say no. You don't have to give a reason. You don't have to explain yourself.

If you're offered alcohol or another drug, you can suggest an alternative: "I think I'd rather have a soda" or "I'd rather not" or something like that. Or you can simply say, "No, thanks."

Choosing to do something that is wrong may be fun for a brief period of time—but it will always catch up with you. There's *always* a price to pay.

If you've already fallen to temptation with alcohol or other drugs, know that Jesus (who faced many temptations too) understands completely and wants you to talk to him and tap into his power.

> For we do not have a high priest who is unable to empathize with our weaknesses, but we have one who has been tempted in every way, just as we are—yet he did not sin. Let us then approach God's throne of grace with confidence, so that we may receive mercy and find grace to help us in our time of need.

Hebrews 4:15–16

As an example of the power of faith to help you make the right choice, think about Moses. As a young man, Moses was tempted to do many wrong things, but he chose not to.

Everybody's *Not* Doing It

At a point in your life (maybe it's already happened), someone will challenge you to do something with the words, "Everybody's doing it."

The temptation might come in the form of shoplifting, going too far sexually, or trying drugs or alcohol. But no matter what the temptation is, know this fact: everybody is *not* doing it.

When it comes to alcohol, studies show that nearly 60 percent of twelve- to seventeen-year-olds have never had a drink. Although some girls have said yes, most girls are saying no.

Experimenting with alcohol is dangerous, and trying other illegal drugs can be even more dangerous. It can even kill you! Taking somebody else's prescription pills, huffing, or trying harder drugs, such as cocaine, can kill a person the very first time they try them.

A very dangerous practice these days is mixing different drugs together — even prescription drugs. At what are called *bowling parties* or *pharm parties*, different pills are thrown in a bowl and people grab handfuls and take them. This is extremely dangerous — people can die after one such party. One expert writes:

> There are dozens of chemicals that can render you friendless, jobless, and despondent — if not outright kill you — all by themselves. That makes taking them together a bit like throwing a mixture of gasoline and fire at your own body. Too much of drug A may cause liver failure, say. Add a little of drug B and it might happen two hours sooner. Toss in drug C, and maybe you'll stop breathing before your liver even gets involved.

So even if someone says "everybody's doing it," when it comes to alcohol and drugs, weigh the consequences, turn to Jesus, and walk away from the crowd.

> By faith Moses, when he had grown up, refused to be known as the son of Pharaoh's daughter. He chose to be mistreated along with the people of God rather than to enjoy the fleeting pleasures of sin. He regarded disgrace for the sake of Christ as of greater value than the treasures of Egypt, because he was looking ahead to his reward. By faith he left Egypt, not fearing the king's anger; he persevered because he saw him who is invisible.
>
> *Hebrews 11:24–27*

Notice, Moses was able to make the right decision by *faith*. His faith became a resource—it strengthened his will to choose right over wrong.

Today, God gives the gift of the Holy Spirit and his Word to guide us to make right decisions. We'll talk more about how to stay strong when tempted in question 34.

We know saying no isn't always easy. But by standing strong, you may find that many of your friends secretly agree with you. They'll likely respect you even more because they know deep down that you are doing the right thing. It may even give them the courage to also say no. You can be an important positive influence in your friends' lives. It takes courage to do what is right even if it seems "uncool." So be brave.

If you continue to get pressured, talk about it with your mom or dad, a teacher, or another trusted adult.

> Wine is a mocker and beer a brawler; whoever is led astray by them is not wise.
>
> *Proverbs 20:1*

A Drop of Friendship

One of our young reviewers, now in college, has the following advice for you:

Though I believe it is a person's choice whether they want to drink alcohol, I've never been sorely tempted to myself.... It's not the smartest of ideas.

When you drink ... your judgment is altered, and it makes people do really stupid things. You don't need to drink to have a good time. I've gone out with friends and had a good time without a single drop of alcohol in my system.

We agree. I (Dr. Mari) have awesome childhood memories. I hung out with my three BFFs almost every weekend. We had sleepovers at each other's houses and spent tons of time talking, laughing, and having fun. We didn't need to have a drop of alcohol to have fun. All we needed was to be together.

Don't drink too much wine. That cheapens your life. Drink the Spirit of God, huge draughts of him. Sing hymns instead of drinking songs! Sing songs from your heart to Christ. Sing praises over everything, any excuse for a song to God the Father in the name of our Master, Jesus Christ.

Ephesians 5:18–20 MSG

QUESTION 30

Sex — part of God's plan?
Are you serious?

God created the universe in a series of steps. And after each step of creation, God said it was all good. But after creating the entire universe, God was not done — the highlight of creation was still missing.

> So God created mankind in his own image, in the image of God he created them; male and female he created them.

Genesis 1:27

After creating a man and a woman,

> God saw all that he had made, and it was very good.

Genesis 1:31

Once he created humans, only then did his entire creation become "very good." Why? Because women and men, girls and boys were the only creatures in the entire universe made in the image of God. God first created the man, Adam. And then he said something surprising: "It is not good ..." (Genesis 2:18).

Why was it *not good*? Everything else in creation was either good or very good. Did God goof up when he made man?

My (Dr. Walt's) daughter, Kate, and I were talking about this once. She smiled and said, "I know why."

"Please go on," I replied.

Kate laughed and said, "Well, it's in the Bible. It says that after God made a man, he said, 'It is not good. I can do better than that.' Then he made a woman."

"What version of the Bible did you get that from?" I asked, laughing.

"The Modern Woman Version," Kate said, joking.

Well, the real reason is *not* that God goofed or that he thought he could do better. Not at all! Men and women are God's beloved creation. Yet God created the man with a very specific need:

> The LORD God said, "It is not good for the man to be alone. I will make a helper suitable for him."
>
> *Genesis 2:18*

God's design is that a man will leave his parents and be united to his wife and become *one flesh* with her (Genesis 2:24). Biblical marriage is a very big deal to God. Jesus emphasized this by saying:

> "Haven't you read ... that at the beginning the Creator 'made them male and female,' and said, 'For this reason a man will leave his father and mother and be united to his wife, and the two will become one flesh'? So they are no longer two, but one flesh."
>
> *Matthew 19:4–6*

God's design for men and women is to have a sexual relationship (to be united and become one flesh) only in the union of marriage where they can then embrace his gift of children. It's all tied together—a man, a woman, sex, and children go together by divine design.

In creating you, God gave your body the ability to carry a child—God's future gift to you and your husband. He designed your womb to carry and nurture a child and to give birth.

Think about it. God created the world in such a way that the creation of people won't happen without the participation of a

Virgin by Grace

A virgin is someone who waits until marriage to have any sexual activity. Unfortunately, some boys and girls are robbed of this choice through sexual abuse. Some young people have been forced into sexual activity by people who are sick, evil, or have bad intentions. Sexual abuse is a crime and a terrible sin. Beyond hurting the child, such abuse hurts God's heart deeply, and God offers those children healing, mercy, and grace.

If this has happened to you, a trained Christian counselor or therapist can help you heal from abuse. Most life-affirming pregnancy centers (also called *crisis pregnancy centers* or *pregnancy resource centers*) have counselors who will talk to you for free. You can find one near you using the URL in our resources list at the back of the book.

Talking to your parent is also extremely important so they can help keep you safe.

If there's been abuse, getting help is very, very important, as is praying and asking God to bring healing to your heart, body, and soul. God can do it.

man *and* a woman. God has trusted us with the best part of his creation — another human being.

This awesome responsibility is a great reason to focus on godly friendships with boys rather than dating while you're still young. In our culture, unless a boy and a girl are very intentional and committed to waiting until marriage to have sex, dating can progress into a physical relationship that neither of them is ready for and both of them may one day regret.

Because physical attraction is so strong, waiting until marriage to have sex can be difficult. It's not impossible, but it takes

Have you ever heard of *secondary virginity?* This is the decision to wait until marriage before having any sexual activity even if you've had sexual activity in the past (whether by choice or through abuse).

The idea is that you can start over *today* regardless of what happened *yesterday.* You can have a fresh start *now* if your choices or experiences robbed you of God's original plan for sexuality.

Although temptation and sin are alive and well in our world, so are God's mercy, forgiveness, and healing. Take him up on his offer of a new life starting right now. Get help from a professional if you haven't already, and believe that God can do great things in you as you trust him with your life, including your sexuality. God promises you hope and a good future.

"For I know the plans I have for you," declares the LORD, "plans to prosper you and not to harm you, plans to give you hope and a future."

Jeremiah 29:11

a strong commitment. If you decide *now* that you will *not* have sex until marriage, it's much easier. Especially since God will help you. He will answer your prayers and help you stay on his best path for your life.

> How can a young person stay on the path of purity? By living according to your word.
>
> *Psalm 119:9*

How cool is that? God gives you the tools you need to use his gift of sex according to his purpose for your life:

1. He gives you the Bible to guide you.
2. He gives you his Spirit to live in you, to teach, and to lead you.
3. He'll give you good Christian friends to walk the path with you.
4. When you are tempted, he'll even give you a way to escape.

So decide *now* and commit not to open the gift of sex until God intends—in marriage—and with the person, the only person, he wants you to have sex with—your husband.

> Marriage should be honored by all, and the marriage bed kept pure.
>
> *Hebrews 13:4*

At your age, rather than focusing on boyfriends and dating, learn instead what makes a good *friend*. Then you will know what qualities to look for in a husband. How else will you know who a boy really is in his heart and soul unless you spend time becoming close friends long before you marry and have sex? You cannot become a soul mate with a guy until you know his soul (mind, emotions, and will/decision making) and his heart (his character—who he really is) deep down. That takes a long time.

This shift in focus away from boyfriends and dating to making great friends will allow you to pray, make good choices, and wait on God's leading for a good husband—a true best friend forever who will love you as Jesus loves you. A man who is a trustworthy companion, your best friend, *and* your soul mate—forever.

Your mom and dad (if you're blessed to have both) can be the key people in your life to help you live this beautiful story. They can help you understand how to make healthy choices in friendships and dating. There are also a lot of great books about dating, courting, and a godly marriage. We've only skimmed over an important topic—one we recommend you learn much more about.

If it is God's will for you to marry and become a mother someday, pray that he will help prepare you for all that's ahead. You can even pray for your future husband to remain pure in heart and body, as you commit to do the same.

> Flee from sexual immorality. All other sins a person commits are outside the body, but whoever sins sexually, sins against their own body.
>
> *1 Corinthians 6:18*

> Flee the evil desires of youth and pursue righteousness, faith, love and peace, along with those who call on the Lord out of a pure heart.
>
> *2 Timothy 2:22*

Have you heard about PAP tests (or *PAP smears*)? These special tests sample cells from your cervix to ensure they're healthy. With this and other tests, doctors can diagnose HPV (human papillomavirus), other sexually transmitted infections (STIs), and cervical cancer—a form of cancer caused by an STI.

Although STIs are quite common, there's only one way to get them—through sexual activity. So you can dramatically reduce your risk of catching *any* STI by avoiding any and all sexual activity until marriage.

Although we hope and pray that you will wait until marriage to become sexually active, we want you to be informed. So let's talk about STIs.

STIs are infections that can be transmitted through *any* sexual activity. This includes any activity in which genital or oral fluids that have the STI germs are spread from a person who is infected to one who is not. You can only get these infections by having sexual activity with someone who's already infected.

Most young girls who begin to have sex *will likely* develop an STI. If you have sex as a young person, you can just about count on becoming infected with something. Why? STIs are very common and can spread easily. And the younger you are, the more likely you are to catch an STI.

Girls often come to our offices with concerns about an abnormal vaginal discharge that started after having sex for the very first time. Even more common, they see us within a year or two of their first sexual encounter and we discover an infection they didn't even suspect. Tears follow, as well as broken hearts.

Even if you only have sexual activity with one person, you can still get one or more STIs from him if he had sexual activity with an infected person. Sadly, we've both had to break the bad news to young girls who caught one of the STIs that can't be cured. When they find out, they're shocked and often say, "But he's been my only boyfriend." They usually have no idea how many other people he'd had sex with already.

Some STIs can cause cancer. Others can keep you from having a baby by causing infertility. Although many STIs can be treated, some of them (like herpes, hepatitis B and C, and HIV [which causes AIDS]) cannot be cured. The best way to "treat" these infections is by *preventing* them.

When STIs lead to symptoms, they can cause burning with urination and/or a vaginal discharge that's thick and gray, brown, yellow, or green. They can cause pain in the lower abdomen and pelvis. If STIs become more severe, they can cause fevers, nausea,

Learn the N.I.C.E. Way to Say No

If you're ever in a situation that goes against your values to remain pure, it helps to plan and even rehearse some ways to say no. The following tips are adapted from the website It's Great to Wait, which you can find with this QR code or the URL in our list of resources:

It's Great to Wait

N Say *no*. Not "maybe" or "later." Set limits and be decisive. If you decide now that you're not having sex until marriage, it will be easier to say no if someone pressures you or tempts you to say yes.

I Follow your "no" with an *"I"* statement: "I'm not going to have sex until I marry." Or "Sex isn't part of my game plan right now." And move on.

C If the pressure continues, *change*. Change the *subject*: "Did you see the game on TV last night?" Or change *who* you're talking to: "I need to go ask Julie something." Or change the *location*: "I'm going back into the kitchen."

E If these strategies don't help, you need an *exit* plan. Leave a bad or unsafe situation *immediately* — no need to be sweet or gracious. Call your parent to get picked up right away. Have a prearranged code phrase that means "Come pick me up. And hurry."

vomiting, a sore throat, rashes, joint pains, and more. They can make you very, very sick.

The most common STIs among young people include HPV (which can cause warts in your private parts and cervical cancer), chlamydia, and gonorrhea. Syphilis, an infection that can even affect the brain, is also on the rise.

Probably the most significant possible consequence of having sex before marriage is pregnancy, since it also impacts another human being—a new life—along with the baby's mother and father and their families. Once a girl starts having periods, even if she doesn't have one every month, she can get pregnant if she has sex!

Although your health teachers at school may tell you that a condom will protect you from some STIs (*not all!*) some of the time, as author Pam Stenzel so wisely said, "There is not a condom in the world that can protect your heart, your reputation, your character, and your values."

Shut That Door

When an STI causes symptoms or damage to your body, we call it a *sexually transmitted disease* (STD). The problem with STIs is that, very often, girls (and boys) don't even know they have them. Here's what happens.

Let's say boy A has the STI called *chlamydia* and doesn't know it, since he has no symptoms. He meets girl B and they have sexual activity, and she gets infected with chlamydia. They don't even have to have sexual intercourse — they may just be touching or kissing each other's genital areas and can spread some STIs like that.

In any case, girl B now has chlamydia and doesn't even know it. She could get symptoms from it, like a yellowish or green discharge or burning with urination. But many times, there are no symptoms.

A month goes by and boy A and girl B break up. They haven't had treatment for their STIs because they don't even know they're infected. Three months later, girl B meets boy C, and they engage

You have some powerful weapons in the battle against STIs: (1) You have the spiritual tools God gave you, and (2) you have your brain and the ability to make good choices.

You can avoid all STIs by choosing to wait on a sexual relationship until marriage *and* by marrying a man who committed to wait for you long before he even met you.

More and more teens and young adults are choosing to live with sexual integrity. This means (1) making choices that keep you pure *now* and (2) waiting for sexual activity until marriage.

in sexual activity. Now boy C, though he never even met boy A, has the same STI, because girl B passed it from one to the other.

Boy C meets girl D. They start making out and end up having sex. She too gets chlamydia, though she has no idea she's carrying the infection. So now four people who don't even all know each other have the STI.

You get the picture. It's not pretty, but this is exactly what happens. We see it in our offices every single day. When it comes to STIs, having sexual activity with one person means you're having sex with everyone he's ever had sex with. Yech!

The revolving door of sex and STIs can be avoided with a simple choice: Shut that door. Have *no* sexual activity of *any* type with *anyone* until marriage. All the public health authorities agree this is the best plan. It's also the plan designed by your Creator. But it's up to you to shut the door to STIs and the heartache and physical consequences they bring.

Dressed to Win

Remember the story about Adam and Eve — how God dressed them after they sinned? Well, God dresses you, too, during your spiritual battles to help you do the right thing and not mess up. He's given you a special uniform that you can put on:

> Therefore put on the full armor of God, so that when the day of evil comes, you may be able to stand your ground, and after you have done everything, to stand. Stand firm then, with the belt of truth buckled around your waist, with the breastplate of righteousness in place, and with your feet fitted with the readiness that comes from the gospel of peace. In addition to all this, take up the shield of faith, with which you can extinguish all the flaming arrows of the evil one. Take the helmet of salvation and the sword of the Spirit, which is the word of God.
>
> Ephesians 6:13–17

Our advice? Don't take off God's special clothing — ever. Check out the following sites with your mom or a trusted adult to learn more about living a pure life *every* day. You can find links to each with the URLs in our resources list at the back of the book:

- True Pink
- TeenSTAR Program
- Abstinence Clearinghouse
- Best Friends Foundation
- Legacy Institute
- True Love Waits

Jesus said:

> "Blessed are the pure in heart, for they will see God."

Matthew 5:8

Nurturing a pure heart and mind will help you keep your body pure. It will also grow your relationship with God, who is the key to all purity. If you make a mistake, by the way, he is the one who forgives you and can help you get back on track.

The good news is that the majority of girls and boys graduating from high school these days have *not* had sexual intercourse. And that majority is growing year by year, as young people learn the truth about and the wisdom of saving *all* sexual activity for marriage. When friends say, "Everyone's doing it," you can say, "No, they're not. *Most* boys and girls are not."

Of those who have sex as teens, three out of four regret that decision and wish they had waited. You can choose to keep yourself pure and preserve all sexual activity until marriage. Not only will you be following God's plan for sexuality, but you'll also avoid the many emotional, spiritual, relational, and physical consequences of these dangerous and costly infections.

Remember the huge responsibility you've been given as a young lady, and protect your gift, your body, and your soul by choosing to live with sexual integrity. You'll be glad you did.

QUESTION 31

Talk to my parents about sex? Are you crazy?

Most parents know that at some point they need to talk to their daughter about love, sex, and her relationships with boys. But most parents say this is not always an easy topic to bring up. For some parents, it's downright stressful!

If one of your parents has not approached you to talk about these things, it could be that he or she is just as nervous about discussing it as you are. Your parent may even be more nervous. So if you feel embarrassed, know you're not alone. It's normal to be a bit apprehensive, shy, and nervous.

We want to make these conversations easier and more meaningful for all of you. We have some ideas to help you start talking about this with one or both of your parents. And if your parent(s) cannot or will not do this, then we'd like to recommend ways for you to pick a trusted Christian woman to talk to.

Now, we're not talking about a onetime "birds-and-bees" talk. We recommend ongoing discussions about sex and sexuality starting now that will continue for years (yeah, it's that important). These conversations should include topics like these:

- What it means to live according to God's Word
- God's gift and plan for sex and sexuality
- How and when to date a young man
- How to apply this information and these principles to your life
- How to choose good friends to help you keep your commitments

As we talked about earlier, the Bible teaches that God designed sex and gave it to married couples as a gift to enjoy. It's a good and wonderful gift. After all, it's from the Creator himself. It's *his* divine design.

As he does with every gift he gives us, he provides some clear rules or boundaries for using the gift of sex. This is an amazing and good thing. Some people think God's rules are meant to keep them from having fun, but that's not true. They're meant to keep you safe—and healthy. God sees sexuality as a beautiful gift, and he loves you enough to tell you how to use it.

Think of it this way. If you're a musician and someone you love gives you a beautiful, fragile, and expensive violin, you'd be a fool to use it as a hammer or baseball bat, right? It would completely ruin it.

Well, your sexuality is an incredibly beautiful, fragile, and precious gift from your Creator. Use it very carefully and wisely. Value and protect it as the treasure it is.

Now, a special note for you girls being raised by a single dad—especially those of you whose mother is no longer with you.

First, three cheers for your dad. Being a single parent is one of the most difficult jobs in the world. He needs your full support, obedience, love, trust, and prayers.

Second, your father can teach you what it means to be treated properly and respectfully by a boy. After all, he once was a boy, he went through puberty, and he can give you some wise advice and warnings about how to dress, how to act around boys, and how to stay safe.

Fun Learning About Sex — Really!

Many ministries offer day or weekend retreats that help moms and daughters start talking in fun and creative ways. Here are the ones we like the best. You can find some links using the URLs in our resources list at the back of the book.

Secret Keeper Girl (for tweens) and Pure Freedom Live (for teens) have live events around the country. You can even go with your mom and your best friends and their moms.

Ideas for mother-daughter weekends away can be found in Family Life's Passport2Purity. These could be some of the most memorable weekends of your life. One of our reviewers noted:

> Although Passport2Purity was originally designed to be done by a mother and daughter, my husband and I took our daughter, age thirteen, away for a special weekend to do this program together. Despite our initial concern that it might be awkward for her to discuss some of these issues with her dad present, it turned out to be such a wonderful addition to have my husband there to communicate the male perspective on the importance of his daughter's purity.

Still, girls are typically most comfortable talking to a woman about sex and sexuality. So if your mom's not around, talk to your dad about choosing a special trusted Christian woman with whom to talk about all this. It may be an aunt, a female youth pastor, an Awana leader, a coach, or some other godly woman you admire and respect.

Another important thing about sex: don't believe everything you see on TV and in the movies. And watch out for books that target tweens and teens but teach you lies about love and sexuality.

Biblical Blueprint for Sexual Integrity is a DVD series designed by the Legacy Institute for parents and their child. The series provides the biblical framework for healthy relationships and an understanding of the divine design of men and women. It will help your parents understand how to explain what it means to be a godly woman.

The Legacy Institute also has a resource called Relationships With Integrity, which has materials for every grade and is ideal for youth groups or small group settings. You might really enjoy going through this series with some of your close Christian friends.

Other great resources to help you understand God's design for your body and sexuality include *Theology of the Body for Teens* and *Theology of the Body for Teens: Middle School Edition.*

Last but not least, we like a Bible study for thirteen- to nineteen-year-old girls called *True Beauty.* This study is designed to teach you what it means to be truly female and truly beautiful. Each chapter teaches you about God's plans in a refreshing and fun way, allowing you and your friends to learn together. Some of the topics you'll talk about include identity, beauty as a gift from God, clothing that reflects true beauty, living whole and balanced lives, nobility, kindness, and much more.

The Talk

For decades, when a parent sat down with a daughter to discuss sex for the first time, it was simply known as "the talk." The problem is that not a lot of parents and daughters are *talking* about sex these days.

Studies show that teens most want to hear about sex and sexuality — believe it or not — from their parents. But that's not what usually happens. Most girls learn about sex through their friends and the media (TV, movies, magazines, social media, videos or DVDs, songs and music channels, the Internet, and porn sites or magazines). Not a great classroom!

The trouble is that what you learn about sex through those sources is usually *not* the best information. Much of it is misleading, a fair amount is just plain wrong, and some of it is meant to harm you or to lead you to make decisions you will regret.

To truly understand and appreciate sex, you have to consider what God says about it in his Word. Since he invented sex and gave it to you as a gift for the future, don't you think he might have a thing or two to say about how to best receive and enjoy this gift?

Research shows that girls who know and live out what the Bible teaches about sex have a more satisfying, fun, and healthy sexual relationship with their future husbands. So we recommend that any talk or talks you have on this topic take place with your mom or dad, or a mature Christian woman, and always include God's Word.

When it comes to your sexuality, make sure to get your information from the best sources you can find—which will usually be your parents (or another trusted Christian female), books like this one and others we recommend, and God's Word.

> Keep your father's command and do not forsake your mother's teaching. Bind them always on your heart; fasten them around your neck. When you walk, they will guide you; when you sleep, they will watch over you; when you awake, they will speak to you. For this command is a lamp, this teaching is a light, and correction and instruction are the way to life.
>
> *Proverbs 6:20–23*

QUESTION 32

Is there a monster in my computer?

Like many girls your age, you probably leaf through teen magazines sometimes. You may look at pictures of pop stars and keep track of their concerts and shows. You may even follow some of them on Twitter or other websites.

Unfortunately, many of these magazines or websites go over the top, and some of them are downright crude. They show pictures of young artists and teen celebrities half naked, wearing just underwear or very provocative clothes. Though this is inappropriate, it's become a normal part of our culture.

Such sexual images are now a part of every girl's life. You literally cannot avoid them. They are in almost every magazine, TV show, and movie, and they're plastered on billboards along many roads. They are everywhere.

Ninety percent of girls your age, those eight to sixteen years old, say they've seen sexual pictures or videos online. In other words, if you're a tween or young teen who spends time on the Internet or texting friends, you're at a high risk of being exposed to sexual images.

When images are sexually explicit (showing private parts or sexual activity), we call them *pornography*, or *porn*. Although looking at these images might seem like harmless fun, it can actually be very dangerous. This is especially true of the super-graphic images on some Internet sites and pop-ups.

The people who make money by hooking others on these images use the Internet as a weapon. You may end up on a site with inappropriate content you weren't even looking for. As you try to get out of it, you realize you're stuck on that awful page. The site has traps built in to keep you there called *mousetrapping*. When you try to click off to leave, a new pop-up appears with even worse images, and the cycle goes on.

If this ever happens to you, stop looking at the images and either power off your computer or use keyboard shortcuts rather than your mouse to click off. Then go find a parent and tell them what happened. Together, you can keep this from happening again.

Mark Kastleman wrote a book about pornography titled *The Drug of the New Millenium*. He says that the chemicals the brain releases when people view sexual images are so intense that experts say they're the most powerful drugs ever known.

You may wonder why this is so dangerous. Here's why. Looking at sexual images, especially if it continues, begins to *change* your brain chemistry, creating a powerful addiction that is tough to break. That's why Kastleman calls porn a powerful drug.

Besides harming your mind, watching sexual images misses the mark of God's best intentions for you. God knows how dangerous this is for your mind *and* heart.

There *Is* a Monster in Your Computer

Looking at sexual images may seem different than staring into the eyes of a dangerous, grotesque, massive monster. But at its core, pornography is a monster that can be hard to control.

If you think porn isn't a worldwide problem, think again. Pornography is a monster with only one goal in mind — to control you and change your view of God's amazing gift of sex. And this monster is aimed right at you.

A U.S. government commission found that the porn industry actually targets twelve- to seventeen-year-olds. Makers of porn know that if they can hook you when you're young, they may have a customer for life.

One expert said showing pornography to teens is like giving crack cocaine (a super-addictive drug) to a drug addict. Their addiction can be extremely hard to break. Sadly, nearly one-third of teens watch pornography often, and nearly every teen has seen at least one pornographic image.

If you have never looked at sexual images on your computer, don't think you're weird or that you're missing something. In fact, we applaud you. You're keeping your mind clean and clear of destructive and disturbing images.

When it comes to pornography, think about it as a monster. Stay away from it. Run from it. Don't think you can chain it up in the basement of your mind. It can still break free and hurt you. Instead of digging around in places on the Internet where you shouldn't go, strive to walk a clean path and honor God with what you put into your mind.

And if you do have a problem with pornography, don't wait to tell a parent or trusted adult. By being open and honest about your secret now, you can start the healing process and kick this monster out.

The number of girls affected by pornography is soaring. One in three kids under ten has been exposed to porn online, and three out of four teens will see a porn image before age eighteen. For most girls, porn is not something they go looking for online, but it's easy to come across these images if you're not careful.

Girls who get hooked on porn say they feel worthless and degraded by their habit. They also say it affects their relationships with others. So remember, the decisions you make now will make a difference for years to come. If your friends are into this and try to get you to join in, choose to guard your heart and mind, and say no.

Don't believe the lie that this is just a problem for guys. That is simply not true. And remember, it helps to look at things through God's eyes—especially when choosing what to look at or listen to.

Sexual immorality (sexual sin) covers many activities that the Bible says are wrong—and you should work hard to avoid them all. Some girls may think, *It's just a picture, or it's just a chat room on the Internet. I didn't actually do anything physically. Therefore, it's not wrong or sinful.*

Except for one thing. Jesus said:

> "You have heard that it was said, 'You shall not commit adultery.' But I tell you that anyone who looks at a woman lustfully has already committed adultery with her in his heart."
>
> *Matthew 5:27–28*

Some girls say, "Guys are gorgeous; they're hot—private parts and all. I'm just admiring God's creation. It's like looking at Michelangelo's naked statue of David. It's art, right?" Sounds innocent enough. Except for the fact that God created that man for his wife to admire and stare at and enjoy—not you.

Also, viewing sexual images can become addicting. Sounds crazy, right? Like all addictions, it starts small but can grow into an ugly monster. And once a girl starts viewing sexual images, she is much more likely to begin acting out sexually. In other words, what goes into your eyes and your mind will affect what you do—your actions.

One of our young female reviewers struggled with this problem for years. She wrote:

> I think the most important thing a girl can do if she is already ... drawn to porn is to reach out. It is so hard, because you feel alone and ashamed and weird, but the more it stays in your mind, the more dangerous it is. So if you can talk to your parents, great. If that is too hard, finding someone older or someone you know will be patient with you is crucial. Also, I think emphasizing to do something now rather than later is important. The longer you wait to stop, the more difficult it is.

We think it is critical that you tell a parent or trusted adult if you're struggling to stop looking at sexual images, since it can affect every area of your life, including your friendships and your schoolwork. Your parents can help find a professional counselor for you to talk to who can help you learn what to do.

Many women who are addicted to sexual images began viewing porn *before* high school. So remember, the decisions you make now will impact the rest of your life.

Now you know why parents set up rules about the kind of TV shows and movies you can watch and which Internet sites you may visit. Certain shows and movies are rated as inappropriate for your age for good reasons—watching them can steal your innocence and harm your mind and heart.

Protect yourself by being choosy about what you allow yourself to watch—whether on TV, DVDs, video games, magazines, or the Internet. Even some commercials are just too much sexually. And guard what you allow yourself to listen to, especially music that plays alongside sexual images like you may have seen on MTV or YouTube.

Bad Apples

We hope your parent has taught you that your private parts are private. No one has a right to touch or see your private parts without your and your parent's permission. No one.

However, people with bad intentions may want to try. Sometimes these people are coaches, teachers, church leaders, Scout leaders, or other youth leaders. We don't want to scare you — most church and youth leaders and teachers are moral and devoted to God, to you, and to their work. But there are a few bad apples in each of these categories. Those bad apples first earn your trust and your parent's trust. And then, when no one's around, they may try to take advantage of you or a friend.

One report found that one in fourteen girls in fifth to eighth grades had been sexually abused by a teacher or coach. For high school girls, the number was one in nine. And these bad people know that most of the girls they abuse will not tell anyone. They use threats and scare the girls to keep them silent. Again, we don't want you to be afraid of all adults in your life — we just want you to know about a real and serious problem that you or your friends may encounter.

No one has found a surefire way to keep these bad apples away from young girls. So you and your friends need to be watchful. You need to know how to protect yourselves and stay safe.

If someone tries to see, photograph, or touch your private parts — or wants you to touch their private parts — forcefully say no and leave. Scream it as loud as you can if you have to! Get away from them. Run to a safe place, and immediately tell your mom or dad or someone in authority, like your principal or a cop or security guard.

Not only will you save yourself from a potential bad guy, but you'll likely save many other girls too.

If TV or Internet programs are causing you problems, turn them off. Choose what you allow to influence your mind, your heart, and your daily thoughts. Ask yourself these questions:

- Would I watch this particular TV show, movie, or website if Christ was in the room?
- Is what I'm doing drawing me closer to God and strengthening my relationship with him or harming it?

Your answers to these questions will help you make wise decisions about what you listen to and watch.

There's one more danger to keep in mind. Looking at porn and visiting chat rooms on the Internet can expose you to *real* bad guys—sexual predators—people who are there to try to take advantage of you or hurt you. So do not ever communicate in chat rooms through IMs, email, or in any way. This is just one more reason to stay away from all that!

As we mentioned in question 28, we suggest that families keep *all* electronic devices, especially those with Internet access, in the living room, family room, or another common room in the house. That way the screen can be seen by anyone in the area. This helps keep the whole family safer and more accountable.

Ask your parents about Internet filters and accountability software to keep your computers safe—we suggest some of our favorites in our resources list at the back of the book.

Also, if porn or a chat room tempts you, consider getting rid of Internet access for a while, and tell your parents and your older siblings so they can help you too.

Throw away any sexually explicit music, magazines, books, or videos you might have and stay away from friends who are into that. Look for a mature Christian woman and some good friends who can hold you accountable and whom you can call if you're tempted.

Remember, don't chat online or exchange messages with *anyone* you haven't met in person, regardless of who they *claim* to be. And if a boy or girl you know tries to message you with sexual images or topics, click "ignore" or "hide" and tell a parent. The best approach is to "unfriend" or block anyone who sends sexual images, since it will probably happen again if you don't.

Your thoughts and actions are important to the Lord—and critical to your future. They will shape the woman you will become. That's why the Bible teaches:

> Whatever is right, whatever is pure, whatever is lovely, whatever is admirable—if anything is excellent or praise-worthy—think about such things.
>
> *Philippians 4:8*

Choose to fill your mind with thoughts of the Lord and what he is doing in your life. As a follower of Jesus, you are not simply to avoid these images; you are to run from them.

> Don't let anyone look down on you because you are young, but set an example for the believers in speech, in conduct, in love, in faith and in purity.
>
> *1 Timothy 4:12*

> Take captive every thought to make it obedient to Christ.
>
> *2 Corinthians 10:5*

If sex is so great, why should I wait?

The time will come to fall in love and explore the wonderful world of romance — when you're older. Until then, of course you'll be curious, and you may find yourself scoping out boys at times and giggling about it with your girlfriends.

If you start to get very interested in boys and get tempted to act on it physically before God's timing for you is right, it will help to have a plan. It helps so much to make up your mind *now* about how you want to live your life.

So decide now to enjoy being a girl — having good friends and being a good friend. Decide now to spend your time and focus your energy on planning for a good future. Decide now not to have to worry about sexually transmitted infections, teen pregnancy, and the many complications that come from getting involved in sexual relationships outside of God's will.

And remember this important truth. You don't need to have a boyfriend to be someone's special girl. You're *already* someone's special girl. You are God's special girl. You are your parents' special girl. And you are your future husband's special girl.

God has such great plans for your life. He wants you to have a good life, and one of the ways he wants to protect you is by helping you live a pure life in every area—including your sexuality.

Sex *binds* a couple together in physical, emotional, *and* spiritual ways. Having sexual activity with someone other than your husband can cause feelings of guilt and shame. Why? Because God designed sex as a wonderful gift that is meant to be enjoyed within marriage. And deep down, most boys and girls know this is true.

Besides the physical act, sex is an *intimate, spiritual* act where two people "become one," and it's not to be taken lightly. When you have sex, you give a huge part of yourself—your body, heart, and soul—to another person. Doing this outside of marriage can have lasting, painful consequences affecting (1) your physical body, (2) your mind and emotions, and (3) your relationship with the person with whom you had sex, your parents, your friends, your future husband, and God.

Think of it like this. When you have *any* form of sexual activity, it's like giving a piece of your heart away to the other person. Do this too much and pretty soon you'll have little of yourself left and less to offer your future husband.

Do you want a husband who will commit his entire life and his entire heart to you? Of course. That's the only kind of man to whom you should consider giving your whole self. You want a man who will wait for you, just as you commit to wait for him to share the precious, God-given gift of yourself.

Without a doubt, waiting to have sex until marriage can be difficult! Every girl will have her sexual nature awakened, often around puberty. One day you're happy enough walking around the mall chatting with your girlfriends. The next day, you suddenly notice every cute boy who walks by. You wonder if he noticed you. You think about going over to meet and talk to him. You tell your girlfriends, and you all check him out and giggle.

This is all normal and can be fun for sure. Yes, do have fun getting to know your girlfriends and boys too — we're all so different. Having good boy and girl friends will help you understand people and your world better. It will also enrich your life.

Risky Business

Here are some of the risks of getting involved in a sexual relationship outside of God's plan:

SEXUALLY TRANSMITTED INFECTIONS (STIs)

- Of the 18.9 million new cases of STIs each year, nearly half are among fifteen- to twenty-four-year-olds.
- Human papillomavirus (HPV) is very common among fifteen- to twenty-four-year-olds who have sex. This virus can cause cancer of the cervix and mouth and painful warts in the private parts.
- Teens, especially girls, are much more susceptible to STIs than adults. That means it's easier for teens and girls to get infected with an STI when exposed to it.
- Some STIs can cause infertility, making it difficult to get pregnant later on when a woman wants to start a family.

TEEN PREGNANCY

- Each year, almost 750,000 young women ages fifteen to nineteen become pregnant.

So enjoy being young following God's plan for your life, and save yourself from the hassles and pain that can come from the wrong relationship at the wrong time. Sex is for later. It's for marriage. It's a gift for you and your future husband. It's also God's plan for bringing new lives into the world.

Choosing to wait until marriage to have any sexual activity helps build a much closer relationship with your future husband—a marriage that's built on trust and love. And that's one important reason why it pays to wait.

- Ten of every 100 babies born in the U.S. have teen parents.
- Teen mothers and fathers are more likely to experience depression, anxiety, single parenthood (splitting up), less education, poverty, and homelessness.
- Children born to teen mothers are more likely to experience health problems, abuse, neglect, poverty, and incarceration (being sent to jail).

TEEN ABORTION

- There are usually more than 200,000 abortions every year among fifteen- to nineteen-year-olds.
- More than one in four pregnancies among fifteen- to nineteen-year-olds ends in abortion each year.
- Most girls and women who have an abortion later experience guilt, shame, and regret similar to *post-traumatic stress disorder* (PTSD), the stress reaction that follows traumatic events. They can also develop severe infections and many other physical, spiritual, and emotional consequences, like depression, poor self-esteem, and guilt.

Accountability Partners

Good friends with similar values and beliefs can help you stay on target, follow God's ways, and make good choices throughout your life. For example, if your close friends are all committed to waiting for a sexual relationship until marriage, it will be easier for all of you to follow through if you have each other. If one of you is tempted, the others can step in to remind her why it's important to stick with God's plan.

Your parents, trusted teachers, and good friends — as well as knowing God's Word — will help you with every choice, like staying away from alcohol and drugs and keeping your mind, heart, and body safe and pure.

A young woman on our review panel wrote:

I can't overemphasize the importance of pursuing relationships with Christian friends. Mine were great. My best friend and I paired up as accountability partners in high school. We then knew we were there as a support for each other but also knew that we could call each other out in love if we were struggling with something. It was so great because someone who was dealing with similar things as me was there to help me through rough times.

Another wrote:

A group of my Christian friends and I made a covenant to be accountability partners when we were in middle school. We agreed to talk to and check on each other often. We agreed to pray for each other. We agreed to ask each other the hard questions about relationships, sex, and sexuality. But most of all, we agreed to be there for each other at all times — 24/7/365. Remaining sexually pure in our culture is never easy. But walking this path with good friends made it so much easier.

It's been just over twenty years since we all became best friends and accountability partners. The last one of us is getting married this summer. We were all able to walk the aisle, sexually pure, because of the help of our Lord and our friends.

> For the LORD will be at your side and will keep your
> foot from being snared.
>
> Proverbs 3:26

Our Purity Ring

One of our book reviewers shared this story with us:

Once I made a commitment to God and to my future husband to be sexually pure until marriage, I began to wear a purity ring on the ring finger of my left hand. When I got engaged, I began to think about the ring I wanted to buy for my husband — his wedding ring.

After thinking and praying about it, I came up with an idea. I talked to a jeweler who helped me design this really cool ring. What the jeweler did was take my purity ring and build my future husband's ring around it.

From the outside it looks like a normal man's wedding band. But when he takes it off, he sees my purity ring on the inside. So it's my ring, stretched out, that is against his finger.

So my wedding ring was a double gift to him — not only my commitment to him on that day, but also a commitment I had made to him long before.

There is a time for everything, and a season for every activity under the heavens.

Ecclesiastes 3:1

QUESTION 34

I want to make wise choices, but how do I stay strong when tempted?

As you grow older, you will face more and more peer pressure. At times, you may consider doing something that could harm you, like smoking, drinking, experimenting with drugs, looking at sexual images, or having sex before marriage. So how do you stand firm when tempted? And how do your choices affect your faith and your relationship with Jesus?

Curiosity is natural and normal. It's normal to wonder about trying a cigarette when you see other kids smoking. It's normal to think about sex when you're bombarded by images every day on TV, in magazines, on the Internet, and even in school. Temptations exist all around you, and they will be there every day of your life.

Being tempted simply means we're human. But the more you learn, the better prepared you will be to make wise choices. Being aware of what's out there can give you discernment, or the ability to use good judgment. Discernment gives you a gut-feeling kind of reaction that helps you determine if something you want to do is right or wrong, or if a situation should be completely avoided. The conscience God gave you also helps you, as does knowing God's Word.

Think about what is important to you right now. How do you want to live? How do you want others to think of you? Do you want to be thought of as a hardworking athlete? A good student? A caring and considerate person? Do you want to stay away from drugs and alcohol? Do you want to be sexually pure until marriage? Deciding ahead of time how you want to live will help you stand strong, even when your friends disagree with you.

As a Christian, your body is a temple, a way to worship God, and God wants you to remain pure. Does this mean that if you mess up God won't forgive you? Absolutely not. But several Truths may help you when temptation strikes.

Truth 1

God may test you. He may allow trials to purify and strengthen you, but he will never lead you into sin. In our culture, people commonly blame their mistakes on peer pressure, leaders, parents, upbringing, genetics, the mailman, their dog, their little toe — whatever. As long as you look for someone or something else to blame, you will have a tough time fighting temptations.

> When tempted, no one should say, "God is tempting me."
> For God cannot be tempted by evil, nor does he tempt anyone.
>
> *James 1:13*

Jesus was tempted in every way, just as we are, and he suffered when tempted. So he knows what it's like, and it's good to have him as our defender.

> For this reason [Jesus] had to be made like [us], fully human in every way, in order that he might become a merciful and faithful high priest in service to God, and that he might make atonement for the sins of the people. Because he himself suffered when he was tempted, he is able to help those who are being tempted.
>
> *Hebrews 2:17–18*

Truth 2

Everyone faces temptation. None of us is tempted in some new or unique way. While we are each completely unique, the temptations we face are basically the same ones that have confronted all people throughout history.

> No temptation has overtaken you except what is common to mankind.
>
> *1 Corinthians 10:13a*

Truth 3

The Bible tells us that when we are tempted, God won't let us be tempted more than we can stand. He will always provide an escape route.

> And God is faithful; he will not let you be tempted beyond what you can bear. But when you are tempted, he will also provide a way out so that you can endure it.
>
> *1 Corinthians 10:13b*

The tricky part is choosing to follow that escape route, which could mean turning off the computer or avoiding certain books, movies, or friends. Sometimes escaping can mean literally running away.

Yes, this can be easier said than done. But there are steps you can take to escape temptation — besides running away.

1. Pray. When tempted, quickly pray to God about what you're experiencing. These on-the-spot, lightning-quick prayers allow you to ask your Father in heaven for grace, wisdom, and strength to avoid the temptation—and to take the way of escape he has provided.

> "Watch and pray so that you will not fall into temptation. The spirit is willing, but the flesh is weak."
>
> *Matthew 26:41*

2. Read Scripture. No matter what happens in your life, the Bible gives you a guide to live by. God's Word gives us rules and advice to help in every situation. Even though the events described in the Bible happened thousands of years ago, its words of wisdom still apply today.

> Your word is a lamp for my feet, a light on my path.
>
> *Psalm 119:105*

> You guide me with your counsel.
>
> *Psalm 73:24*

Plus, memorizing and reciting Scripture can help during times of temptation. Think about your favorite Scripture when your thoughts turn negative.

> How can a young person stay on the path of purity? By living according to your word.... I have hidden your word in my heart that I might not sin against you. Praise be to you, Lord; teach me your decrees.... I meditate on your precepts and consider your ways. I delight in your decrees; I will not neglect your word.
>
> *Psalm 119:9, 11–12, 15–16*

The Word of God is powerful. Jesus used Scripture to defeat Satan when he tempted Jesus in the desert.

3. Avoid temptation in the first place. Don't put yourself in situations where you know you will be tempted. That greatly increases your chances of messing up. Since you're too young to date, even if you're just hanging out with guys, be careful who you spend time with and where you go. And make sure your parents know who you are with and where you are. Always go out with a group. Also, avoid friends who encourage you to watch movies or go places you know your parents wouldn't allow — or tell those friends in advance you won't participate.

On several occasions, Christ told his disciples to pray that they might not fall into temptation. He knew that prayer makes a huge difference.

> "This, then, is how you should pray: 'Our Father ... lead us not into temptation, but deliver us from the evil one.'"
>
> *Matthew 6:9, 13*

4. Encourage one another. Since we are all tempted in similar ways, we can help, support, and learn from each other. As Christians, God wants us to help each other and build each other up in our faith (Ephesians 4:15–16). Having a group of girls who can talk and pray together can really help you avoid specific sins that so many young women fall into.

Here's what one of our teen reviewers said about friends:

> During your teen years, your friends are a huge part of your life, so choose them wisely. You go to school with them for seven hours a day and they make a huge impact on your life whether you realize it. Choose friends who will uplift you in the good and bad times and challenge you in your walk with the Lord.

5. Confess. When you fall, pray and ask for God's forgiveness and for strength to avoid the temptation the next time. Tell a parent or trusted friend about your mistake. Ask her to pray for you. Confession clears your heart and mind.

Make this your common practice: Confess your sins to each other and pray for each other so that you can live together whole and healed. The prayer of a person living right with God is something powerful to be reckoned with.

James 5:16 MSG

Finding good friends and mentors will help you stand strong when facing the temptations common to the teen years. Think about what makes friends good. Do they encourage you or put you down? What do you talk about together, and what do you watch and read? Where do you hang out? Is your friend a Christian?

Think about friendships like strong trees. So what does a tree have to do with encouraging others and finding people who will help you avoid temptation? A lot actually. Coastal redwoods grow to huge heights—the tallest one grew higher than a football field is long—but these trees have shallow root systems. Their roots only go four to six feet deep and spread out more than one hundred feet. These redwoods are able to survive terrible winds and rains by growing close to each other and interlocking their roots to strengthen one another.

By supporting each other, redwoods live thousands of years and become mighty trees.

Good friends help each other grow stronger in their faith. They also make life a lot more fun. So put down roots with some Christian girlfriends who share your goals and values and grow some lives that stand out for Christ.

"A new command I give you: Love one another. As I have loved you, so you must love one another."

John 13:34

It's better to have a partner than go it alone. Share the work, share the wealth. And if one falls down, the other helps, but if there's no one to help, tough!

Ecclesiastes 4:9–10 MSG

Congratulations. You got through thirty-four key questions about your body and puberty. Can you believe how much you've learned? Imagine trying to navigate the difficult path of adolescence without all this information. We've been so happy and blessed to walk this path with you.

You probably have other questions we haven't answered. But by now we hope your relationship with your parents or another trusted adult has given you a safe person to whom you can bring any question or concern.

Now we want to cover one last question every young girl has: When will I be a woman?

Becoming a woman is not about a specific date. It doesn't magically happen when you get your first period or when your breasts begin to grow. It certainly doesn't happen when you get that first pimple. It is a process. You are, right now, becoming a woman. The goal is to grow each day into the young woman whom God created you to be.

Our culture defines your purpose in strange ways. We hope by now you understand and believe that you are much, much more than how you look. We've talked about our culture's obsession with a not-so-beautiful outer "beauty" that's shallow on the inside and leaves girls feeling empty, thinking they don't measure up. Our prayer is that you will not fall for those lies.

Instead, we pray that you will see yourself through the eyes of your Creator, the one who knows and loves you like no one else. This is, in fact, every girl's dream — to know that she is loved just the way she is. And you are! You are precious and loved just as you are.

Once you choose to become a follower of Jesus, once God is the God of your heart, you become a temple of God's Holy Spirit. You are what the Bible calls a jar of clay. Yes, that's right. This is a metaphor for a remarkable truth about the source of your inner beauty and spiritual strength — God's life within you!

> But we have this treasure in jars of clay to show that this all-surpassing power is from God and not from us.
>
> *2 Corinthians 4:7*

Like clay, you are fragile on the outside but house a treasure on the inside. Nowhere in the Bible are you called to focus excessively on the jar. Instead, you are told to guard your *heart* — above all else.

> Above all else, guard your heart, for everything you do flows from it.
>
> *Proverbs 4:23*

Jesus' emphasis always moves you from focusing on the outside to the inner life. He wants you to focus on your heart.

> "The LORD does not look at the things people look at. People look at the outward appearance, but the LORD looks at the heart."
>
> *1 Samuel 16:7*

I (Dr. Mari) recently bought a devotional book for tweens to read with my daughter. I looked forward to reading a chapter a night with her and learning together. When I gave it to her, she leafed through it briefly and went right back to playing. I could almost hear her thoughts: *I'm playing now, Mami. Maybe later.*

That night, when I entered Hannah's wonderland to tuck her in, I found her reading. She said she couldn't put down her new book. "You didn't wait for me," I said, and she smiled.

Hannah didn't wait for me the next day either, or the next day. She read the whole book that week. Like you, she was thirsty for the truth. She wanted to learn more about life and what's important for girls to know about themselves and about God.

For weeks, we talked about the stories in the book. We soaked our feet, had tea parties, and laughed a lot. Months later, she still brings up the stories she read, which gives us another chance to chat about life. I cherish those moments with her—your loved ones do too.

Just this week we had another special moment, this time at the mall. After getting some cool nail polish, I noticed Hannah looking away when we walked by store mannequins in their underwear. She did what she'd learned in one of the stories she read. She was guarding her eyes and her heart.

I'm not sure exactly what she was thinking, but as we walked on, she suddenly said, "Mami, I am a faith girl that's dressed in God." Even at a very young age, girls can learn to think with God's mind, focusing not on their bodies but on their hearts.

Her beautiful (and true) statement reminded me of what she'd said months earlier while surrounded by Disney princesses: "Faith dresses me and makes me beautiful in God's eyes." She is so right.

As a young woman, you are beautiful in God's eyes. He loves his special and unique creation—you. And when you let his goodness and love shine through you, you look even more beautiful.

We hope and pray you'll think about true beauty for the rest of your life. A beautiful, godly woman brings glory to God and displays his character to everyone she meets. And this is precisely what you are called to be and what we pray you are becoming—one day at a time.

When you choose to live according to God's ways, he helps you live a life that's pure, holy, and true. When you offer yourself back to your Creator, you begin the greatest adventure of all. A life of knowing, following, and loving God is better than any fairy tale—it is the adventure of a lifetime.

We invite you to stop reading for a moment to think and pray about these questions:

- Who am I?
- Whose am I?
- Why does it matter?

Consider jotting some thoughts in your journal. Your answers are important because the way you see yourself comes through in the things you say and do—in the way you live.

For the rest of your days, choose to nurture your inner life with God's love and truth, focusing on your heart, and the rest will take care of itself. Focus on being a courageous, committed, and faithful woman of God—like Esther. Choose to be obedient and surrender to God's plans—like Mary. Choose to serve others—like Mother Teresa. All three of them became women of God when they were very young. So can you.

Find God's path for you in your gifts and godly passions—those things you love to do. And focus on growing the garden of your spirit, bearing its fruit of love, joy, peace, patience, kindness, goodness, faithfulness, gentleness, and self-control.

Such a harvest spreads Jesus in the world and makes your heart glad. Self-respect is beautiful. Kindness and goodness are beautiful. Thoughtfulness and gentleness are beautiful. Your inner beauty will shine through in the way you treat yourself and others.

You may be thinking, *This sounds great, but it's hard to do all the time.* We agree. Living like Esther, Mary, or Mother Teresa is not easy, but it *is* possible with God's help and the help of those who love you.

Continue to use your journal to work through your emotions, thoughts, and feelings, and share with your mom and trusted adults as you continue to grow up. Stay close to godly role models and friends. No one has all the right answers, and neither will you, but God does. His wisdom will keep you safe.

Respect and treat yourself with the same kindness and gentleness that you'd want to offer to the friends you love. Identify and use your God-given gifts—this will bring you joy and enrich your life and those around you. And make going to church a priority. Although it may not always be fun, staying in church means you continue to hear God's Word and learn to apply it to your daily life. This will help deepen your faith and keep you close to God.

Ask for help when you need it. God blessed you with parents, teachers, role models, friends, and family. Many people love you and want God's best for your life. Talk to your parents and siblings when you need help or have questions—that's what they're there for.

Embrace the gifts of your femininity and sexuality, and keep yourself pure as you await the blessing of marriage. Be smart. Don't go with the crowd. Don't blend in with those who don't follow Jesus. Be different. If you want to find a crowd to follow and imitate, choose a group that honors God and demonstrates godliness.

Although this way of life may *feel* lonely at times, you are *not* alone as you choose the path of righteousness—of thinking and doing right things.

Throughout the world, young men and women are speaking out for godliness, truth, and a pure life. Join them. Become a voice for purity and godliness. Become a voice of hope to your generation. Like Mary and Esther, you can choose to be courageous and live dressed in the beauty of God's love.

> Therefore, if anyone is in Christ, the new creation has come: The old has gone, the new is here!
>
> *2 Corinthians 5:17*

> So then, just as you received Christ Jesus as Lord, continue to live your lives in him, rooted and built up in him, strengthened in the faith as you were taught, and overflowing with thankfulness.
>
> *Colossians 2:6–7*

FINAL WORD
FOR DAUGHTERS
AND PARENTS

When my (Dr. Walt's) daughter, Kate, turned six years old, my father called her to wish her a happy birthday. I beamed like any proud dad, and then Kate turned to me. "Pops would like to speak with you," she said as she handed me the phone.

"Congratulations." my father declared.

"For what, Dad? What did I do?"

"It's Kate's one-third birthday."

That made no sense, so I pointed out, "She's six years old, Dad."

"Yes, but one-third of your life with her is over."

One-third? You mean I was one-third of the way through raising this little pipsqueak of a girl who favored coloring books and story time? It didn't seem possible. She was so tiny. But I instantly understood what my father was saying: at eighteen, she would leave home — my child-rearing days would be over, and Kate's childhood days would be past.

You may be wondering what this has to do with you. Well, if you're twelve, two-thirds of your time with your parents as a child is gone.

And for you, parents, your child-rearing days are two-thirds complete.

You're both more than halfway through. You're rounding the clubhouse turn, and the finish line is in sight. Just like any race, though, the homestretch can be the toughest ground to cover.

For you tweens and teens, if you haven't figured it out by now, what matters most is not the *things* you get from your parents.

You need *your parents* — their love, their cheerleading, their advice and guidance, their steering and teaching, and, most of all, their time and prayers.

Every tween and teen needs her parents to spend quality time with her. It's critical to learn that quality time can only occur within quantity time — a concept I learned when I read a book written by my friend, family physician Richard Swenson. In *Margin: Restoring Emotional, Physical, Financial, and Time Reserves to Overloaded Lives*, Dr. Swenson explains how the health of families is being destroyed by parents (especially dads) who leave little room in their schedule for their kids.

I was blessed to read this book just as God used my dad to urge me to spend more time with Kate and her brother, Scott. Back then, my day started with early hospital rounds, followed by eight or more hours of patient care in the office and then evening hospital rounds. This schedule left little margin for me to spend time with my wife or children.

My father's encouragement and Dr. Swenson's book inspired me to do something about that. I met with my medical partner, and we agreed to a new work schedule: On Tuesdays and Thursdays, I'd stop seeing patients at 2:00 p.m. so I could meet one of our children at the bus stop by 3:00 p.m.

Tuesday afternoons and evenings were for Kate, and Thursdays were for Scott. My time with Kate involved helping her with homework, and then we'd take walks, read together, or go get a milk shake. Sometimes we'd just sit for a while and have long talks about anything and everything.

I had a blast with this time set aside for my children. And so did they. I came to know and love my kids in a new way, which never could have happened any other way. I learned that quality time occurs only in the midst of quantity time. In other words, to have many special moments together, you need to spend time together regularly.

When Kate was nineteen, I was invited to introduce Dr.

Swenson at a medical conference. Kate was with me, and when she heard that Dr. Swenson was there, she asked to introduce him. Here's what she said that afternoon:

> Ladies and gentlemen, when I was a little girl, my daddy read a book that Dr. Swenson had written. The book was called *Margin*. In that book, my daddy learned that if he wanted me to be as healthy as I could be physically, emotionally, relationally, and spiritually, he would have to spend some time with me—a lot of time.... So my daddy took time away from work and spent every Tuesday afternoon and evening with me.... I'm embarrassed to tell you that I don't remember a lot of the gifts my parents have given me during my childhood, but I will never forget the memories I have from those days with my daddy.

Then Kate turned to Dr. Swenson and said, "Dr. Swenson, I want to thank you for teaching my daddy. Because of what he did, I will never be the same."

So our final word to you is this: Create some margin—open up space for each other in your life—and spend precious time *together*.

Highly healthy girls will spend time with their moms and their dads. Parents who give their kids both love *and* time help them become healthy and whole. Moms and dads, if your parents didn't give you this gift, you have a chance to break the cycle with your children.

And, girls, if you feel like you don't get enough time with your parents, pray about it and pray for them. When the time is right, have a heart-to-heart chat and let them know how you feel. Let your mom or dad know how much you want to and need to spend more time with them.

Believe us, it will be worth it.

> Let us not love with words or speech but with actions and in truth.

1 John 3:18

Last, thanks for allowing us to be a small part of your journey from girlhood to womanhood. Our prayer for you is that you mature into a wonderful woman of God—that you choose to develop and practice the character traits of a woman of integrity—traits that must be learned and practiced. God's life in you—his wisdom and grace—will help you grow into the woman he created you to be.

As you grow into all God has planned for you, choose to follow his ways. Remember that God's rules and limits are designed to protect you—because he loves you. So choose to do what's right even when parents and teachers and police officers aren't around.

God's love calls you to honor and obey your parents and teachers. As a young woman of character, do all you can to get along with your parents. And thank them for working hard so you can have a home, clothes, food, and everything you need.

A great way to thank your parents is by understanding that food, clothes, furniture, water, and electricity cost money. So don't waste them. Take care of your clothes and your room. Be sweet to your siblings and help care for your pets and home. Be a good steward of all things entrusted to your care.

As a growing, young woman of God, be honest, loyal, and trustworthy. Be a good friend and serve others without expecting thanks or a reward.

Nurture a pure heart that will help you wait until marriage to have sexual activity. Commit to a pure life now and do everything you can to wait for and then remain married to one person for life.

Commit to read the Bible to hear God speak to your heart, and speak to him through prayer and quiet time every day. Attending church will also bring you closer to your family, your church family, and to God.

Finally, get to know yourself—your heart, feelings, and dreams—and be genuine, sharing your feelings and thoughts with trusted friends. Learn to respect others' feelings and beliefs. And be authentic. God didn't make you to be someone else. He made you to be you!

How does a young girl do and become all of this? Simply by walking with Jesus through *each* day, letting him be the God of your heart and choices, listening to him, and learning from him.

Still, every woman of God will make mistakes, and it's great to know that God's heart is full of grace for you. He loves you so much just the way you are. And he gives you his Spirit to guide and lead you. As Paul writes:

> Be on your guard; stand firm in the faith; be courageous; be strong. Do everything in love.
>
> *1 Corinthians 16:13–14*

A life spent following God is full of "love, joy, peace, patience, kindness, goodness, faithfulness, gentleness, self-control; against such things there is no law" (Galatians 5:22–23, NASB). As you devote yourself to being a woman after God's own heart, your Creator—the God of the universe—is on your side. You will be blessed, and you will be a blessing to many.

> Trust in the LORD with all your heart
> and lean not on your own understanding;
> In all your ways submit to him,
> and he will make your paths straight.
> Do not be wise in your own eyes;
> fear the LORD and shun evil.
> This will bring health to your body
> and nourishment to your bones.
>
> *Proverbs 3:5–8*

ACKNOWLEDGMENTS

We're thankful to a volunteer panel of expert advisers who spent considerable time reviewing this book and have, with their corrections, advice, and wisdom, made it much more accurate and reliable:

Psychologist

Arlyn Brunet, PhD (psychologist, San Juan, Puerto Rico).

Authors/educators/youth specialists/pastoral professionals

Carrie Abbott (family/youth educator, Kenmore, WA); Carrie Archual (youth specialist, Indianapolis, IN); Jennie Bishop (author, Daytona Beach, FL); Mary Margaret Collingsworth (youth specialist, Franklin, TN); Robert Fleischmann (pastor/theologian, Hartford, WI); Leah Kilcoin (pastoral professional, Matthews, NC); Jessica Lubbers (youth specialist, Mechanicsville, VA); Yvette Maher (pastoral professional, Colorado Springs, CO); Mark Merrill (attorney and family/youth specialist, Tampa, FL); Susan Merrill (family/youth specialist, Tampa, FL); Diane Passno (family specialist, Colorado Springs, CO); Kate Ritz (youth specialist, Colorado Springs, CO); Jessica Sanders (youth specialist, Denton, TX); Angie Schlossberg (educator, Wynantskill, NY); Lynnette Simm, EdD (educator, Prosper, TX); Becky Wood (pastoral professional, Baton Rouge, LA).

Medical professionals

Ruth Bolton, MD (family physician, Madison Lake, MN); Freda Bush, MD (obstetrician/gynecologist, Jackson, MS); Vicki Clark, CMA (Certified Medical Assistant, Colorado Springs, CO); Patti

Francis, MD (pediatrician, Moraga, CA); Lauren Franklin, MD (family physician, Niceville, FL); Darla R. Grossman, MD (family physician, Evansville, IN); Ed Guttery, MD (pediatrician, Fort Myers, FL); Susan A. Henriksen, MD (family physician, Glen Rock, PA); Leanna Hollis, MD (internal medicine, Blue Springs, MS); Paula Homberger, PAC (physician assistant, Colorado Springs, CO); Julian Hsu, MD (family physician, Centennial, CO); Pearl Huang-Ramírez, MD (family physician, Kissimmee, FL); Kim Jones, MD (pediatrician, Los Altos, CA); Gaylen M. Kelton, MD (family physician, Cicero, IN); Mark Lytle, MD (pediatrician, Birmingham, AL); Nicole McVay, RN (nurse, Tulsa, OK); Mary Anne Nelson, MD (family physician, Cedar Rapids, IA); Ann Park, MD (women's development coach, Tampa, FL); Kent Petrie, MD (family physician, Avon, CO); Amarillys Sojo, MD, (Swansea, IL); Patty Stitcher, RN (nurse, Littleton, CO); Alice Ko Tsai, MD (obstetrician/gynecologist, New York City, NY); Paul R. Williams, MD (pediatrician/neonatologist, Pisgah Forest, NC); Laurel Williston, MD (family physician, Tulsa, OK); Joanne Woida, PT (physical therapist, Orlando, FL); Jean Wright, MD, MBA (pediatrician/health system executive), Mint Hill, NC; Gentry Yeatman, MD (adolescent medicine, Tacoma, WA).

Mothers

Valerie Alexander (Birmingham, AL); Carey Clawson (Larkspur, CO); Zanese Duncan (Norcross, GA); Idaliz Good (Kissimmee, FL); Shannon McLaughlin (Celebration, FL); Kathy Norquist (Eagle Creek, OR); Lois Osborn (Larkspur, CO); Jenny Rapp (Falmouth, MA); Sally Zaengle (Greene, NY).

Young women

Harper Alexander (Birmingham, AL); Julia Campbell (Troutdale, OR); Brianna Clark (Colorado Springs, CO); Grace Clawson (Larkspur, CO); Christianna Bishop (South Daytona, FL);

Meredith Clawson (Larkspur, CO); Kelly Gutrich (Tinley Park, IL); Lindsay Henriksen (Glen Rock, PA); Jessica Jones (Los Altos, CA); Annie McVay (Tulsa, OK); Arlyn Moret-Brunet (San Juan, Puerto Rico); Hannah Osborn (Larkspur, CO); Gracie Roberts (Moraga, CA); Courtney Runn (Austin, TX); Casey Lee Sheffey (Lake Mary, FL); Jennifer Sojo (Tallahassee, FL); Hannah Woida (Orlando, FL); Bethany Wright (Mint Hill, NC).

In particular, Carrie Abbott; Carrie Archual; Freda Bush, MD; Robert Fleischmann; Darla R. Grossman, MD; Diane Passno; and Pearl Huang-Ramírez, MD, spent significant time helping us with their extensive review of early manuscripts of the book. Thanks to Andrea Vinley Jewell, Patrick Dunn, and Barb Larimore for over-the-top editorial assistance. Appreciation is due to Ned McLeod and D. J. Snell for legal and contract assistance. We're also grateful to Kim Childress and the team (including Cindy Davis, Guy Francis, and Greg Johnson) at ZonderKidz for the trust they extended in asking us to write this book.

But we're most thankful to God for calling us into the unmatched privilege of being his children. We pray that this book will bring honor and glory to him, his name, his kingdom, his word, his Son, his Spirit, and his church.

Walt Larimore, MD, Monument, CO
Amaryllis Sánchez Wohlever, MD, Orlando, FL

December 2013

RESOURCES

Question 1: What does it mean to be healthy?

God's Design for the Highly Healthy Teen. http://tinyurl.com/arfzmdz
10 Essentials of Happy, Healthy People: Becoming and Staying Highly Healthy. http://tinyurl.com/amcbhzy
God's Design for the Highly Healthy Teen Assessment. http://tinyurl.com/ao4wnxu

Question 3: Why are there things about my body I just don't like?

My life is but a weaving ... adapted from Grant Colfax Tullar's poem "The Weaver" http://tinyurl.com/l2zkdhl

Question 5: Am I growing — or is the ceiling dropping?

Stature-for-Age Chart:
- http://tinyurl.com/n92u7sh

Predicting your adult height:
- http://tinyurl.com/ygfe2o
- http://tinyurl.com/264hutv

Question 7: Do I really need calcium for my bones?

Best Bones Forever. www.facebook.com/bestbonesforever

Question 8: Makeup, hairstyles, clothes — what makes me beautiful?

Mother Teresa. http://tinyurl.com/s6k5p

Question 9: Why do I look so different from the girls I see on TV?

Photoshopping examples:
- http://tinyurl.com/yfbeeka
- http://tinyurl.com/bb25wuw

Magazines we recommend:
- *Sisterhood* (for teens). http://tinyurl.com/azz82nc
- *Discovery Girls* (for tweens). http://tinyurl.com/yzqmj2h

- *SHINE* (for nine- to fourteen-year-olds) and *Sparkle* (up to age ten). http://tinyurl.com/b3v488q

Nicole Clark's DVD and workshops. http://tinyurl.com/nzc3rwy

Leah Darrow. http://tinyurl.com/asolcfd

Question 10: Should I go on a diet?

National Eating Disorders Association. http://tinyurl.com/b7h35h

BMI percentile calculator. http://tinyurl.com/4tazduc

Become TV-free:

- http://tinyurl.com/yqj9u5
- http://tinyurl.com/azsnzus
- http://tinyurl.com/b38z6sh

Question 11: What can I do if I'm overweight?

Learn to read nutritional labels. http://tinyurl.com/cw948

SuperSized Kids Test activity and nutrition assessment test. http://tinyurl.com/bjoz2ju

Eight-Week Family Fitness Plan. http://tinyurl.com/12b21b4

Meet Families who have used the eight-week plan. http://tinyurl.com/bklelw4

Level 2 (Advanced) Eight-Week Family Fitness Plan. http://tinyurl.com/bxabe94

SuperSized Kids: How to Rescue Your Child from the Obesity Threat. http://tinyurl.com/bgbosgh

Question 13: How do periods work, anyway?

Ovulation video. http://tinyurl.com/ye8rkco

Question 18: Can my moods be dangerous?

Eating disorders information:

- http://tinyurl.com/a9argd6
- http://tinyurl.com/6w3skv2

Question 20: Why do I sweat? It makes me feel like a boy.

"Tanning" Your Smelly Feet:

- The People's Pharmacy. http://tinyurl.com/ajttkee
- Dr. Oz. http://tinyurl.com/ak59qq7

Question 21: What's the big deal about modesty?

Pure Fashion. http://tinyurl.com/bz6qwcz

Question 22: Clothing, thoughts, and good choices — what's the connection?

The Modesty Survey. http://tinyurl.com/aames7x
Saige Hatch's Modesty Club. http://tinyurl.com/bcbqn8w
8 Great Dates for Moms and Daughters. http://tinyurl.com/ncbvh2k
Secret Keeper Girls' Truth or Bare Fashion Tests. http://tinyurl.com
/krpt5hd

Question 23: Nails, makeup, and hair — how much should I care?

Curly Girl: The Handbook. http://tinyurl.com/cmwca6c
Hair Styling Tips and Tricks for Girls. http://tinyurl.com/bfsu5dl

Question 28: Social media is fun, but how much is too much?

What Would Jesus Text? WWJTXT? http://tinyurl.com/a87hc5x
Plugged In media reviews. http://tinyurl.com/as28qzv

Question 29: What if my friends want to try alcohol, drugs, or dangerous games?

The choking game:
- http://tinyurl.com/arx6fs5
- http://tinyurl.com/aczkemr

Question 30: Sex — part of God's plan? Are you serious?

It's Great to Wait. http://tinyurl.com/4zvbatd
Virgin by Grace. Find a counselor near you:
- Heartbeat International's Option Line, (800) 712-HELP or http://tinyurl.com/alldskm
- Focus on the Family, (800) A-FAMILY
True Pink. http://tinyurl.com/bbpfe96
TeenSTAR Program. http://tinyurl.com/b5462te
Abstinence Clearinghouse. http://tinyurl.com/l9nt7x
Best Friends Foundation. http://tinyurl.com/a5l3nfe
Legacy Institute. http://tinyurl.com/bbpfe96

Question 31: Talk to my parents about sex? Are you crazy?

Secret Keeper Girl. http://tinyurl.com/a7v36v3
Pure Freedom Live. http://tinyurl.com/9wunuuy
Family Life. http://tinyurl.com/b8oa85
Passport2Purity. http://tinyurl.com/acwllde
Biblical Blueprint for Sexual Integrity. http://tinyurl.com/abc5c63
Legacy Institute. http://tinyurl.com/ay3h48g
Relationships With Integrity. http://tinyurl.com/b5mqqp8
Theology of the Body for Teens. http://tinyurl.com/b397pjh
Theology of the Body for Teens: Middle School Edition.
    http://tinyurl.com/6nn556w
True Beauty Bible study. http://tinyurl.com/bbpfe96

Question 32: Is there a monster in my computer?

The Drug of the New Millennium. http://tinyurl.com/bcx4x6q
Internet filters and accountability software:
* Bsecure Online. http://tinyurl.com/ya8vx64
* Netintelligence. http://tinyurl.com/bcktmtx
* Covenant Eyes. http://tinyurl.com/nrf8tc
* X3watch. http://tinyurl.com/c6avbrv

Final Word for Daughters and Parents

Richard Swenson, *Margin: Restoring Emotional, Physical, Financial, and Time Reserves to Overloaded Lives* (Colorado Springs: NavPress, 2004). http://tinyurl.com/ay7qjxs

Faithgirlz Journal
My Doodles, Dreams, and Devotion

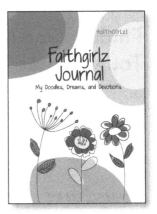

Just between you and God looking for a place to dream, doodle, and record your innermost questions and secrets?

You will find what you seek within the pages of the Faithgirlz Journal, which has plenty of space for you to discover who you are, explore who God is shaping you to be, or write down whatever inspires you. Each journal page has awesome quotes and powerful Bible verses to encourage you on your walk with God! So grab a pen, colored pencils, or even a handful of markers. Whatever you write is just between you and God.

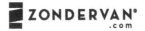

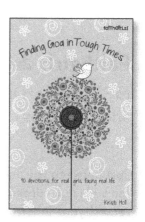
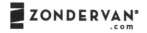

Real Girls of the Bible

31-Day Devotional

Mona Hodgson

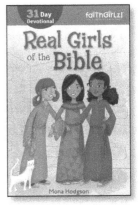

View your world with fresh eyes.

From Faithgirlz comes Real Girls of the Bible, featuring thirty-one stories about real girls from the Old and New Testaments. Just like you, each of these girls had to find her place in the world, and though your worlds are very different, you'll find that many of the struggles were the same—like fitting in and struggling to do the right thing. Each devotion includes Scripture, prayer, Body Talk, and more. With thirty-one days of devotions, discover what real girls from the Bible might have to say about finding your way.

Available in stores and online!

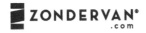

You! A Christian Girl's Guide to Growing Up

Nancy Rue

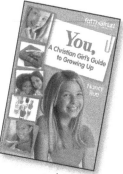

Knowledge is power, girlfriend.

One day you were an easy-going kid, and the next—wham! You're an emotional roller-coaster. Hair is growing in all-new places, and your best friend whispers the word "bra" in gym class.

Discover God's plan for the beautiful, confident, grown-up you!

Everybody Tells Me to Be Myself but I Don't Know Who I Am, Revised Edition

Nancy Rue

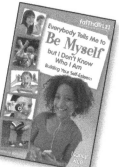

How many times have you heard grown-ups say, "Just be yourself"?

But how can you be yourself when that self always seems to be different—depending on where you are, who you're with, or what you're doing? This book will help you figure out who you really are deep down inside. You'll learn to be the young women God created you to be!

Girl Politics, Updated Edition

Nancy Rue

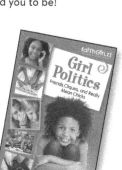

In this revised edition, bestselling author Nancy Rue provides a guide on how to deal with girl politics, God-style.

Girl Politics has all the info on friends, bullies, frenemies, and more, with real-life examples, conversation starters, Internet tactics, and tips to protect yourself—God style—Revised and updated with more examples from real girls, tackling more issues relevant in today's media-driven world.

Available in stores and online!

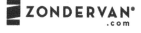

Every girl wants to know she's totally unique and special. These Bibles say that with Faithgirlz! sparkle. Through the many in-text features found only in the Faithgirlz! Bible, girls will grow closer to God as they discover the journey of a lifetime.

NIV Faithgirlz! Bible
Hardcover

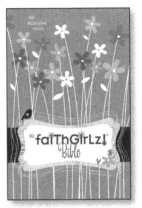

Features include: ✶ Book introductions—Read about the who, when, where, and what of each book. ✶ Dream Girl—Use your imagination to put yourself in the story. ✶ Bring It On!—Take quizzes to really get to know yourself. ✶ Is There a Little (Eve, Ruth, Isaiah) in You?—See for yourself what you have in common. ✶ Words to Live By—Check out these Bible verses that are great for memorizing. ✶ What Happens Next?—Create a list of events to tell a Bible story in your own words. ✶ Oh, I Get It!—Find answers to Bible questions you've wondered about. ✶ The complete NIV translation ✶ Features written by bestselling author Nancy Rue

NIV Faithgirlz! Backpack Bible
Italian Pink Duo-Tone™

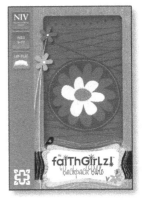

Small enough to fit into a backpack or bag, this Bible can go anywhere a girl does. Features include: ✶ Fun Italian Duo-Tone™ design ✶ Twelve full-color pages of Faithgirlz fun that helps girls learn the "Beauty of Believing!" ✶ Words of Christ in red ✶ Ribbon marker ✶ Complete text of the bestselling NIV translation

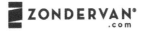

Young Women of Faith Bible, NIV

Susie Shellenberger,
general editor

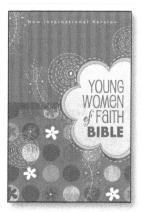

The study Bible that's just for girls!

This Bible is filled with engaging features that will help you learn more about yourself and your relationship with God. Designed to encourage you to develop a habit of studying God's Word, you'll discover how relevant the Bible can be to your everyday life. Weekly studies and many of the side notes are also linked to the women's study Bible, the NIV Women of Faith Study Bible, allowing you and your mom to share God's Word together.

Features include:
- Weekly Bible studies apply biblical truths to life
- Side notes address difficult passages and offer historical and cultural insights
- Journal captures other girls' experiences or struggles along with space for you to record your own
- "I Believe" statements of faith and foundational beliefs
- "Memory Challenges" are verses worth remembering
- "If I Were There . . ." include Bible stories that place you in the Bible character's situation

Available in stores and online!

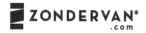

My Beautiful Daughter

What It Means to Be Loved by God

Tasha K. Douglas

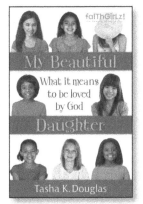

Sometimes You Need a Daddy's Hug.

Every girl wants to be loved by her daddy. But maybe yours isn't around as much as you'd like, or isn't around at all. If so, here's the awesome truth: we all have a Father who loves us deeply, completely, and forever. You'll meet him in this book—through quizzes and real-life stories about girls just like you. Plus, you'll read stories of real women who were able to change the world because of their heavenly Father's love. Discover a Father who loves you, wants to know you, and can help you through anything. He's the most incredible Father ever, and he thinks you're pretty special too.

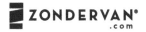

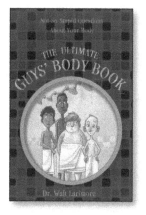
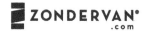